RECENT ADVANCES IN IMMUNOLOGY

RECENT ADVANCES IN IMMUNOLOGY

Edited by

Asuman Ü. Müftüoğlu

Cerrahpaşa Medical Faculty of
University of Istanbul
Istanbul, Turkey

and

Nefise Barlas

Admiral Bristol Hospital
Istanbul, Turkey

PLENUM PRESS • NEW YORK AND LONDON

Library of Congress Cataloging in Publication Data

Main entry under title:

Recent advances in immunology.

"Proceedings of the fifth European Immunology Meeting, held June 1982 in Istanbul, Turkey" — P.
Includes bibliographical references and index.
I. Immunology — Congresses. 2. Immunopathology — Congresses. I. Müftüoğlu, Asuman Ü. II. Barlas, Nefise. III. European Immunology Meeting (5th: 1982: Istanbul, Turkey) [DNLM: 1. Allergy and immunology — Congresses. W3 EU882 5th 1982r/QW 504 E89 1982r)
QR180.3.R43 1984   616.07'9   83-24494
ISBN-13: 978-1-4684-4651-7   e-ISBN-13: 978-1-4684-4649-4
DOI: 10.1007/978-1-4684-4649-4

Proceedings of the fifth European Immunology Meeting,
held June 1982 in Istanbul, Turkey

© 1984 Plenum Press, New York
Softcover reprint of the hardcover 1st edition 1984

A Division of Plenum Publishing Corporation
233 Spring Street, New York, N.Y. 10013

PREFACE

The aim of this publication is to present the up-to-date views of the many eminent immunologists who contributed to the scientific program of the 5th European Immunology Meeting held in Istanbul in June 1982. Recent Advances in Immunology is intended for immunologists both in the basic sciences and in clinical medicine. It provides under one cover an assemblage of information about fundamental problems in immunology and clinical applications.

The book opens with Prof. E.A. Kabat's review of the problems in understanding the structural basis of antibody complementarity. The succeeding four papers deal with the role of macrophages in the various stages of immune phenomena. The first of the two articles on T cells reports a product necessary for suppressor activity and the second describes an analysis of precursors of cytotoxic T lymphocytes. The articles dealing with immunogenetics start with the description of new loci in HLA by Prof. J.J. van Rood and co-workers followed by a paper describing the molecular cloning of H-2 class I genes. Prof. P.J. Lachmann begins the discussion on the genetics of the complement system. There are three stimulating articles on the chemistry and genetics of the complement components and their associations with disease. After a review of artificial antigens and synthetic vaccines, papers on immunomodulation describe strategies for improving immunogenicity, immunomodulation in tumor systems and by xenobiotics.

A report on the technical difficulties and improvements of the human-human hybridoma system links the first part of the book with the clinical immunology papers. The discussion of lymphocyte dysfunctions associated with enzyme defects is followed by three papers dealing with various forms of immunodeficiency. The section on autoimmunity starts with the discussion of T cell regulation in autoimmune diseases. A comprehensive paper by Prof. D. Doniach and G.F. Bottazzo describes the principles of early detection of autoimmune endocrine disorders. The role of autoimmune T lymphocytes in the pathogenesis of myasthenia gravis gives a good example of the cooperation between laboratory and clinical medicine. Finally some of the patho-physiological mechanisms of immediate type hypersensitivity

v

are discussed in three papers: the properties and function of human
IgG short term sensitizing anaphylactic antibody, leukotrienes and
lipid factors and the regulation of imflammatory reactions by
calmodulin.

The contributors deserve all the credit that the meeting may have
achieved in bringing into perspective much new knowledge in the
various fields of immunology. Their cooperative efforts are much ap-
preciated. We are convinced that a book giving the highlights of the
Istanbul Meeting is particulary timely and we hope that it will be
well-received.

Asuman Ü. Müftüoğlu, M.D.
Nefise Barlas, M.D.

CONTENTS

CONTENTS

PROBLEMS IN UNDERSTANDING THE GENERATION

OF ANTIBODY COMPLEMENTARITY

Elvin A. Kabat

The National Institute of Allergy and Infectious
Diseases, National Institutes of Health, Bethesda,
Maryland, and the Departments of Microbiology, Human
Genetics and Development, and Neurology, and the Cancer
Center/Institute for Cancer Research, Columbia University
College of Physicians and Surgeons, New York, U.S.A.

A major problem of the present decade is the elucidation of the
structural basis of antibody complementarity, or, in other words,
what do antibody combining sites of a given specificity look like
and how do the various amino acid side chains make for different
kinds of combining sites (1-3). Intimately related to this is the
question of how the capacity to make these sites is maintained in
the germ line. The genetic basis for the formation of antibody combining sites differs from that of all other proteins with specific
receptor sites such as enzymes, hormones and lectins in that antibody combining sites are formed by two chains whereas other receptor
sites are essentially built of a single chain. It was generally es-
timated that mammals could form about 10^6 antibody combining sites
but since the development of the hybridoma technique (4) this estimate must clearly be low by several orders of magnitude since to
date no two hybridomas making antibody combining sites to a single
antigenic determinant such as $\alpha 1 \rightarrow 6$ dextran have been found to be
identical (5-7).

Let us consider what we know about the structure of antibody
combining sites. As the amino acid sequences of light and of heavy
chains of immunoglobulins were being determined, it became clear
that both the light and heavy chains had a domain structure each
domain having a disulfide bond with a loop of about 55-70 amino
acids and that the antibody combining site was associated with the
N-terminal domain of each chain termed the V_L and V_H domains
(V=variable) respectively (Figure 1). The earliest sequence studies
were carried out on human Bence Jones proteins shown by Edelman and

1

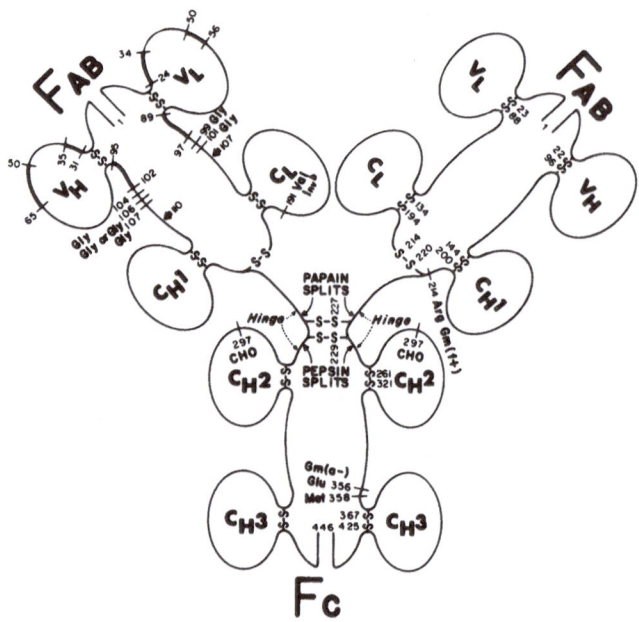

Fig. 1.   Schematic view of four-chain structure of human IgG$_\kappa$ molecule. Numbers on right side denote actual residues of pro-
tein Eu (8,9). Numbers of Fab fragments on the left side
are aligned for maximum homology; light chains are numbered
according to Wu and Kabat (10,11). Heavy chains of Eu have
residue 52A and 82A, B, C and lack residues termed 100A, B,
C, D, E, F, G, H and 35A, B. Thus residue 100 (end of variable region) is 114 in actual sequence. Hypervariable regions and complementarity-determining segments or regions
are shown by heavier lines. V_L and V_H denote light- and
heavy-chain variable regions; C_H1, C_H2, and C_H3 are domains
of constant region of heavy chain; C_L is constant region of
light chain. The hinge region in which two heavy chains are
linked by disulfide bonds is indicated approximately. At-
tachment of carbohydrate is at residue 297. Arrows at residues 107 and 110 denote transition from variable to constant
regions. Sites of action of papain and pepsin and locations
of a number of genetic factors are given. (Reproduced with
the kind permission of Academic Press).

Gally (11) to be the light chains of immunoglobulin; no two human
Bence Jones proteins were found to have identical amino acid sequences in their amino terminal first domains and this led to their
being termed variable regions. The antigenic specificity of Bence
Jones proteins had permitted them to be classified into two classes,
κ and λ and these were ascribable predominantly to amino acid differences in the second or C domain (Figure 1); all κ light chains,

had the same amino acid sequences except for two positions at which Mendelian allelism was shown to occur. The three C-domains of the heavy chain were comparable to the C-domain of the light chain and C-domains were responsible for functional properties of antibodies other than their ability to combine with antigen (13).

As amino acid sequences of light chains accumulated, it was possible by aligning the chains for maximum homology to undertake a statistical analysis of each position in the variable region, using the formula (10)

$$\text{Variability} = \frac{\text{Number of different amino acids occurring at any given position}}{\text{Frequency of the most common amino acid at that position}}$$

to show that there were three regions of high variability, termed hypervariable regions (10) and shown by the heavy portions of the V-domain in Figure 1. It was predicted that the chain would fold so that the combining site would be formed by the three hypervariable regions. Mouse V_λ chains were also sequenced; 12 mouse V_λ chains were identical throughout the V-region and seven variants differed by from one to three amino acids all involving one base change and all but one in hypervariable regions. These were ascribed to somatic mutation (14,15). Similar data supporting somatic mutation were found for some mouse V_K sequences (15). When a sufficient number of heavy chain sequences became available, they too were found to have three hypervariable regions (Figure 2) (11). Hypervariable regions are unique to immunoglobulins and are seen in no other collection of proteins such as the cytochromes etc. (1-3). The inference that the combining site was formed by the three hypervariable regions of each was supported by affinity labeling studies (17) and was completely verified when X-ray crystallographic studies of Fab fragments (18, 19) and of Bence Jones protein dimers or Fv dimers were carried out (20-22) and the hypervariable regions in each instance formed the walls of the combining site (Figure 3); thus these are now termed CDR (complementarity-determining regions) (1), the remainder of the domain constituting a framework (FR) which serves to position the CDR at the tip of the molecule. That the FR of the various proteins are essentially similar has permitted attempts to construct antibody combining sites by replacing the CDR of these structures with the CDR of known antibody molecules. A major limitation of the X-ray crystallographic studies to date is that the determinant for which the site is specific is not known, the two Fab fragments (18,19) being from myeloma proteins and the Bence Jones dimers forming primitive sites in which one V_L region orients like the V_H region (20).

Until X-ray crystallographic studies at high resolution are car-

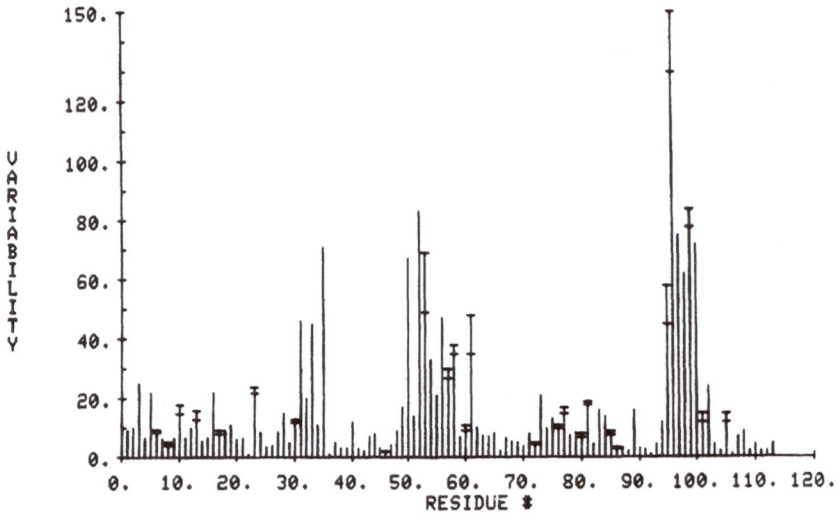

Fig. 2. Variability at different positions for the variable region
of heavy chains. The plot was made by the PROPHET computer
system (16). (From 37).

ried out on an antibody molecule with a combining site specific for
at least one antigenic determinant of defined specificity which
fills the site completely and to see how the determinant is oriented
in the site, progress in understanding antibody complementarity will
be limited. With several or even one such structure rapid strides
can be made.

Antibody combining sites may be mapped immunochemically by determining the structure of the hapten which fits into an antibody
combining site (23). This is accomplished by a variety of methods
which measure the strength of binding directly as an association
constant or by measuring the relative capacity of various haptens
on a molar basis to displace the antigenic determinant from the site.

The reaction between $\alpha1\rightarrow6$ dextran and human antidextran provided
the first system used to measure the size of an antibody combining
site. The isomaltose oligosaccharides ($\alpha1\rightarrow6$ linked) from the disac-
charide to the heptasaccharide were used to inhibit the precipitin
reaction between $\alpha1\rightarrow6$ dextran and antidextran and essentially provided a molecular ruler for measuring sizes of antigenic determinants and antibody combining sites (24-26, see 23). On a molar basis
the best inhibitors were found to be the hexa-and heptasaccharides.
With most antisera, the hepta- and hexasaccharides were equally
potent but with antidextran from one individual, the hepta- was

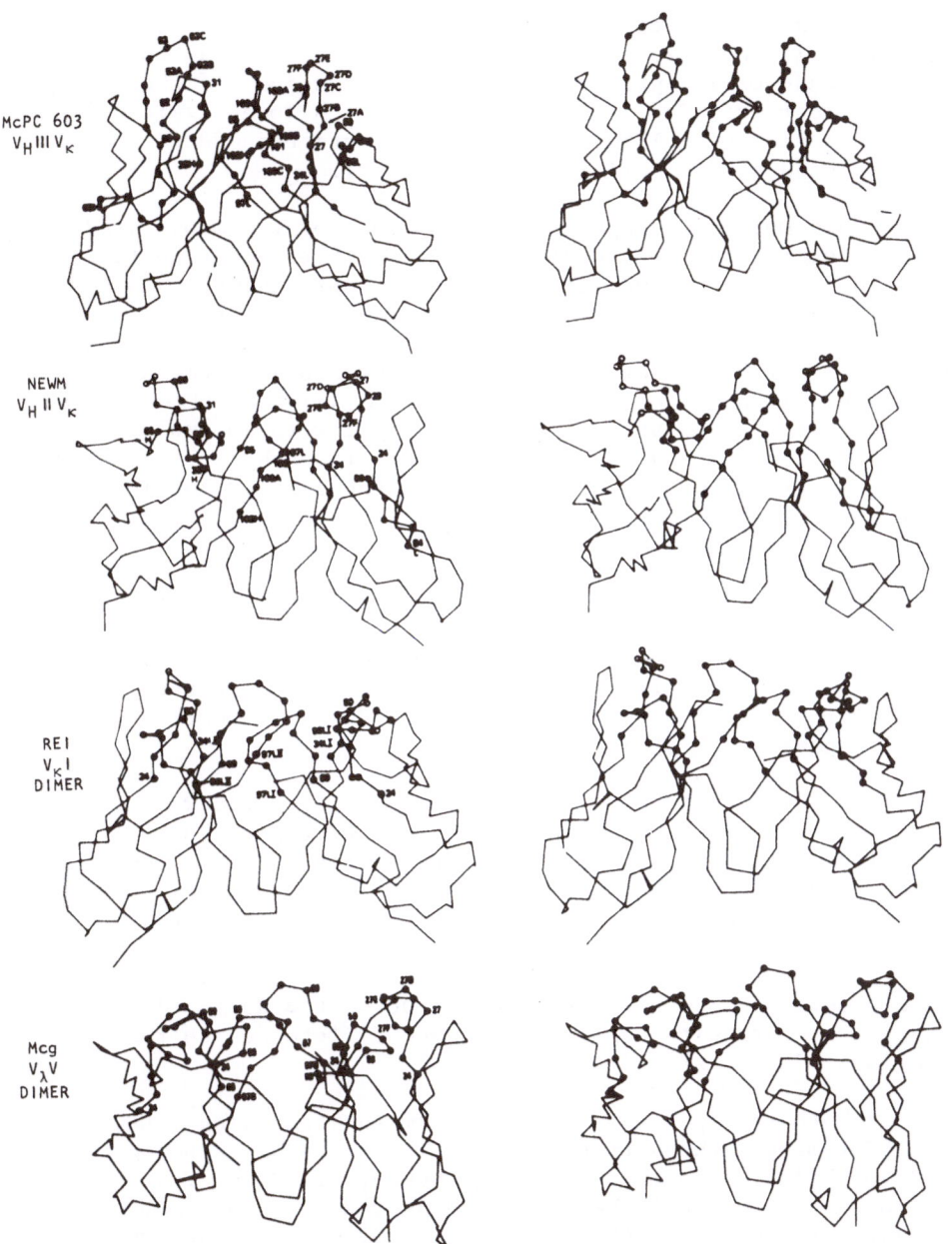

Fig. 3. Stereodrawings of the α-carbon skeletons of the V-regions
         of four of the five proteins studied crystallographically.
         Each protein is in the same orientation. With a stereoviewer
         it is possible to see two adjacent models at the same time
         so that a comparison may be made in three dimensions.

slightly but significantly better than the hexa-; thus establishing
the upper limit for size of the $\alpha 1 \rightarrow 6$ antidextran site as complementary to a hexa- or a heptasaccharide, the dimensions of the hexasac-
charide in most extended form being 34x12x7Å. A lower limit of about
4 to 6 Å was also established and (27) all antigenic determinants
which have been mapped fall within these limits.

When this method was applied to the study of two mouse myeloma
proteins specific for $\alpha 1 \rightarrow 6$ dextran, sites complementary to five and
to six glucoses were found (28), the former surprisingly having an
association constant thirty times higher than the latter. By evaluating the relative contribution of each sugar to the total binding
energy an important difference was seen. The smaller combining site
had a higher affinity for methyl αDglucoside and isomaltose whereas
the larger site showed very little affinity for these two sugars,
significant binding requiring at least the trisaccharide isomaltot-
riose. Moreover the myeloma antibody with the smaller combining site
did not precipitate with a synthetic linear dextran but inhibited
like the pentasaccharide whereas the myeloma antibody with the larger
combining site precipitated with the linear dextran. This allowed us
to infer that the smaller size site was complementary to the ends of
chains with the non-reducing one or two glucoses being held in three
dimensions -e.g., had a cavity type combining site whereas the larger
size site had a groove-type site since it could precipitate with the
linear dextran. Studies with myeloma antibodies to other polysac-
charides supported this distinction (29-31).

Twelve hybridoma antibodies induced in BALB/c mice were found
to have groove type sites in that they were precipitated by linear
dextran (6); six had sites complementary to six and the other six
to seven glucose units; however they differed in affinity constants
and in the relative contribution of each sugar to the total binding
energy (7). Thus all 12 hybridoma antibodies had different combining
sites. Determination of the V-region sequences and X-ray crystallographic studies should provide information on the detailed structure
of these combining sites and how sequence differences correlate with
the various binding affinities.

Since both the V_L and V_H domains form the combining site, it was
natural for many workers to hypothesize that random recombination of
V_L and V_H chains could create a large number of sites. Thus, 10^6
sites could theoretically be generated by random recombination of
10^3 light with 10^3 heavy chains. This is not the case however. With
the 12 $\alpha 1 \rightarrow 6$ hybridoma antidextrans which were obtained from a myeloma
parent which secreted κ chains, it could be shown that the κ chains
from the myeloma parent associated with the heavy chain less well
than did the κ chain from the antibody synthesizing cell (5). In the
most definitive study with six hybridomas secreting anti-fluorescyl
antibody only the six homologous V_L-V_H recombinations were found to
bind fluorescein (32). Thus a major problem becomes to learn what

determines association of a given V_L with V_H in the formation of
antibody combining sites. To date no one has found a heterologous
recombinant which presents a new defined specificity.

In a collaborative study (33) of 12 hybridoma antibodies to
dextran B1355S, a highly branched dextran built of alternating $\alpha 1 \rightarrow 3$
and $\alpha 1 \rightarrow 6$ linked glucoses, it was possible to classify the antibodies
into five groups by quantitative precipitin curves with a panel of
20 dextrans. All of the hybridoma antibodies and two myeloma antibodies J558 and MOPC104E reacted best with three highly branched
dextrans containing the highest proportion of $\alpha 1 \rightarrow 3$ linkages and the
alternating $\alpha 1 \rightarrow 6$ $\alpha 1 \rightarrow 3$ pattern. The classification into the five
groups was based on the number of cross reacting dextrans and the
extent of cross reactivity. Group 1 reacted only with the three
highly branched dextrans and did not react with the other dextrans.
One would have expected all three to have identical sequences in the
CDR. However, the heavy chains differed in all but one residue in
CDR3. This reveals an unsuspected type of antibody specificity which
may further complicate precise understanding of the generation of
antibody complementarity. If the cross reactions involve a subsite
of the antibody combining site, then it would appear that in the
group 1 hybridomas, access to this subsite may be blocked by different amino acid side chains in the CDR; an analogous situation
has been found in the sites of chymotrypsin as compared with elas-
tase. The former site contains two glycines whereas the latter has
valine and threonine which do not permit access of certain chymotrypsin substrates with bulky side chains (34). Another suprising
finding is that members of different groups may differ only by a
single amino acid in the entire V_H domain. This suggests that the
light chains, although λ are contributing to the site complementarity.
There also appears to be some correlation between precipitin group,
the D region positions 96 and 97 (CDR3) and the MOPC104E individual
idiotype (IdI), the two hybridomas and MOPC104E having Tyr and Asp
at these positions being in precipitin group 5. Hybridomas with
IdI(J558) with Arg and Tyr at these positions and J558 are in groups
1 and 3.

If we now consider the remarkable insights which have come from
application of recombinant DNA technology we find that a major change
in thinking has been the result of the discovery of intervening sequences and the splicing out of the primary transcript formed in the
nucleus to give the cytoplasmic mRNA which is translated on the ribo-
some to give the protein chain (35). Immunoglobulin genes show two
unique features: 1. The variable region is assembled from gene segments during differentiation and 2. the joining of the V to the C
region and the switch from one immunoglobulin class to another is
accomplished by splicing out not only of the intervening sequences
but also of the coding sequences between the chain initially synthesized, IgM, and the chain resulting from the switch. The order
of the C-region genes in the mouse has been shown to be $5'-C\mu-C\delta-$

$C\gamma3-C\gamma1-C\gamma2b-C\gamma2a-C\epsilon-C\alpha-3'$ (36). We shall only consider the genes or gene segments involved in the synthesis of the V_L and V_H domains.

In organizing our data base of amino acid sequences in the PROPHET computer (37), we noted that two human $V\lambda$ chains, a $V\lambda II$ and $V\lambda V$ had 21 differences in amino acid composition and yet had an identical first CDR of 14 amino acids (38). A human $V_K I$ and a $V_K III$ had 30 amino acid differences but were identical in CDR3 (39). As there were very few identical CDR, we ordered the FR segments into sets, all members of a given set having an identical amino acid sequence. When each chain was traced from one FR to another (Figure 4) (40), there appeared to be an independent assortment of FR segments. Moreover, FR4 seemed to be independent of the V_K subgroup, since $V_K I$ could be in the same FR4 set with $V_K II$, $V_K III$, or $V_K IV$ confirming earlier observations that V_K subgroups could not be traced beyond amino acid 94 (41). Similar assortment of FR segments of human and mouse $V_H III$ chains were seen and it was subsequently possible to assort the FR and CDR segments of rabbit light chains (42).

The first sequence of a clone containing a germ line $V\lambda$ gene from 12 day mouse embryo had just been reported (43) and it was found to code only through amino acid 96. It was known that the V-region of the secreted adult plasmacytoma light chain extended through amino acid 107 or 108 and from this and the assortment data, it was hypothesized that the FR and CDR were gene segments (minigenes) and that the genes coding for the FR and by implication for the CDR were assembled somatically during differentiation to give an intact V-region. Shortly thereafter two additional clones were found, one from 12 day old embryo coding for amino acids 97-108, termed the J segment, followed by an intervening sequence and the gene coding for the entire C_L region (44). The second from adult plasmacytoma coded for the intact V-region. Thus the assortment data were confirmed; the nucleotides coding for the J segment, with intervening sequences 5' and 3', constituted a minigene. Cloning of embryo mouse V_K chains, showed that there were five J segments (45,46), one of which J3 was a pseudogene, each separated by intervening sequences. Each coded for amino acids 96-108. The intervening sequence after J5 was followed by the C_K coding region. The four functional J_K minigenes were seen to assort independently (47). Sequences of mouse germ-line genes coding for heavy chains showed the presence of four J_H minigenes (48,49) which also assort independently as seen in the five classes of B1355 antidextran hybridomas (33).

Assortment of FR segments of mouse V_K light chains could also be demonstrated at the DNA level (50). A library from mouse myelomas MOPC21 was screened and 28 V-containing clones were isolated which did not hybridize to C or J region probes and were considered to represent unrearranged embryonic V-region genes. These were used in dot blot screening with probes approximately containing nucleotide sequences coding for the different FR segments. All clones hybridized

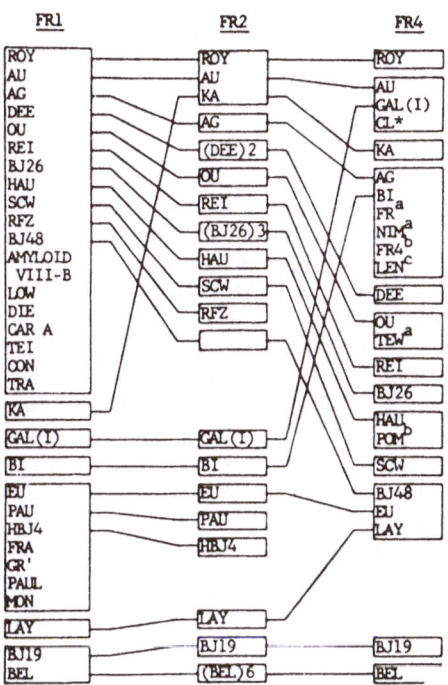

Fig. 4.   Independent assortment of framework sets in human $V_\kappa I$
           chains. Solid circle, cold agglutinin with antiblood group
           I activity; a, human κ light chain subgroup II; b, human
           κ light chain subgroup III; c, human κ light chain sub-
           group IV. (From 40).

to the intact V-region probe. Six hybridized to all probes for FR1,
FR2 and FR3 and probably represent the gene family usually seen by
Southern blotting which is apparently less sensitive than dot blotting. Three clones hybridized only to FR1, 10 only to FR2, and 9 only
to FR3. While these assortment data are consistent with the minigene
hypothesis, sequencing of the clones will be necessary to establish
whether or not they are already assembled in the germ line or whether
they exist as minigene segments.

    When germ line heavy chain genes were sequenced it was noted
that the V-region was coded for only through FR3 (48,49). The four
J segments generally contained nucleotides coding for FR4 plus
several residues of CDR3. However the V and J segments, unlike findings with light chains did not code for the intact chain, segments
coding for from five to 14 amino acids were missing. This segment
was termed the D or diversity segment and the D segments are also
minigenes since they are surrounded by intervening sequences. D minigenes were subsequently isolated (51-53) and found to have signal

sequences of nonanucleotide, a 12 base spacer and a heptanucleotide
5' to the coding sequence and a heptanucleotide a 12 base spacer and
a nonanucleotide 3' by which they can join to the V and J and it has
been proposed that D-D joining may account for the length variations
in CDR3. Four human D minigenes have been identified by hybridization
with a probe containing the signal and recognition sequences (54).
When the coding nucleotide sequences were translated in all three
reading frames into amino acid sequences (55), it was found that the
D2 minigene coded for a segment Ser-Gly-Gly-Ser-( )-Tyr present in
CDR2 (55), residues present in two fractions of Type III antipneu-
mococcal antibody from a single rabbit (56,57,37) (Table 1). A single
V_HIII germ line gene has been sequenced (58) and it was found (55)
that fourteen successive nucleotides matched this D2 minigene also
in CDR2. The probability of this occurring by chance is 1 in 10^8.
A second V_HII germ line sequenced by Rechavi and Givol (unpublished
data) had an exact match of 13 of the same fourteen nucleotides, the
difference being in the first nucleotide. This raises many questions.
Can the D minigene insert into CDR2 as well as into CDR3 by a gene
conversion mechanism? Are there other minigene segments coding for
parts or all of CDR2 and perhaps even of CDR1? Why does the DR minigene account only for a portion of CDR2?

There are several other findings which would be accounted for
satisfactorily by the minigene hypothesis. One of these is that there
are identical stretches of from three to nine nucleotides (59) in
mouse V_K and V_λ chains which mark the junctions of FR and CDR segments and could serve as sites for assortment by gene conversion.
A second is the finding that identical amino acid sequences in FR2
occured in 1 human V_KIV, 21 mouse V_K and 13 rabbit V_K chains. Thus,
this FR2 amino acid segment has been preserved for 80 million years
(60). Nevertheless numerous alternate forms are present but occur
relatively infrequently. If all V-regions exist in the germ line as
contiguous nucleotide stretches coding through CDR3, this preserved
segment would have to occur many times in the germ line and one
wonders why this FR2 segment has been preserved over so long a
period in evolution when it is apparently able to exist in multiple
alternate forms. Many of these alternate forms, especially in the
rabbit were in light chains from antibody molecules (60).

Assortment of FR and CDR segments for the V-region excluding J
and D has been proposed by Baltimore (61) and by Egel (62) to account for the assortment data. If such gene conversion occurs somatically, it would account for the assortment data in a manner effectively equivalent to the minigene hypothesis. If it occurs only
in evolution, the preserved FR2 will require some other explanation.

At present diversity is apparently generated by V-J and V-D-J
joining, by somatic mutation, evidence for which has also been obtained at the nucleotide level (63) and by gene conversion. The role
of each of these mechanisms in generating antibody complementarity

Table 1.   Comparison of nucleotide sequences of CDR2 of a human V_H gene, V_H26, with four human D minigene segments (55).

Amino Acid Residue	Amino Acid	Nucleotide Sequence				
		V_H26	D1	D2	D3	D4
50	Ala	G				
		C				
		T	A	A	A	A
51	Ile	A	G	G	G	G
		T	G	G	C	G
		T	A	A	A	A
52	Ser	A	T	T	T	T
		G	A	A	A	A
		T	T	T	T	T
52A	Gly	G	T	T	T	T
		G	G	G	G	G
		T	T	T	T	T
53	Ser	A	A	A	G	A
		G	C	G	G	G
		T	T	T	T	T
54	Gly	G	G	G	G	A
		G	G	G	G	G
		T	T	T	T	T
55	Gly	G	G	G	G	A
		G	G	G	A	C
		T	T	T	T	C
56	Ser	A	G	A	T	A
		G	T	G	G	G
		C	A	C	C	C
57	Thr	A	T	T	T	T
		C	G	G	A	G
		A	C	C	T	C
58	Tyr	T	T	T	T	T
		A	A	A	C	A
		C	T	C	C	T
59	Tyr	T	A	T		G
		A	C	C		C
		C	C	C		C
60	Gly	G				
		G				
		A				
61	Asp	G				
		A				
		C				
62	Ser	T				
		C				
		C				
63	Val	G				
		T				
		G				
64	Lys	A				
		A				
		G				
65	Gly	G				
		G				
		C				

as distinct from diversity or genetic noise is an area which must
be explored further in the future.

ACKNOWLEDGEMENT

    Aided by grant PCM 81-02321 from the National Science Founda-
tion and grant CA 13696 to the Cancer Center of Columbia University.
Work with the PROPHET computer system is supported by the National
Cancer Institute, National Institute of Allergy and Infectious
Diseases, and the National Institute of Arthritis, Diabetes, and
Digestive and Kidney Diseases and the Division of Research Resources
(contract N01-RR8-2118), of the National Institutes of Health.

REFERENCES

1. Kabat, E.A., Adv. Protein Chem. 32:1-75 (1978).
2. Kabat, E.A., J. Immunol. 125:961-969 (1980).
3. Kabat, E.A., Pharmacological Rev. 34:23-38 (1982).
4. Köhler, G. and Milstein, C., Nature (Lond.) 256:495-497 (1975).
5. Sharon, J., Kabat, E.A. and Morrison, S.L., Mol. Immunol.
    18:831-846 (1981).
6. Sharon, J., Kabat, E.A. and Morrison, S.L., Mol. Immunol.
    19:375-388 (1982).
7. Sharon, J., Kabat, E.A. and Morrison, S.L., Mol. Immunol.
    19:389-397 (1982).
8. Edelman, G.M., Biochemistry 9:3197-3205 (1970).
9. Edelman, G.M., Cunningham, B.A., Gall, W.E., Gottlieb, P.D.,
    Rutishauser, U. and Waxdal, M.J., Proc. Natl. Acad. Sci. U.S.A.
    63:78-85 (1968).
10. Wu, T.T. and Kabat, E.A., J. Exp. Med. 132:211-250 (1970).
11. Kabat, E.A. and Wu, T.T., Ann, N.Y., Acad. Sci. 190:382-393
    (1971).
12. Edelman, G.M. and Gally, J.A., J. Exp. Med. 116:207-227 (1962).
13. Winkelhake, J.L., Mol. Immunol. 15:695-714 (1978).
14. Cohn, M., Blomberg, B., Geckeler, W., Raschke, W., Riblet, R.
    and Weigert, M., in: "The Immune System, Receptors, Signals",
    eds. by E.E. Sercarz, A.R. Williamson, and C.F. Fox, pp. 89-117,
    Academic Press, New York (1974).
15. Weigert, M. and Riblet, R., Cold Spring Harbor Symp. Quant.
    Biol. 41:837-846 (1976).
16. Raub, W.F., Fed. Proc. 33:2390-2392 (1974).
17. Givol, D., Essays Biochem. 10:1-31 (1974).
18. Amzel, M., Poljak, R.J., Saul, F., Varga, J.M. and Richards,
    F.F., Proc. Natl. Acad. Sci. U.S.A. 71:1427-1430 (1974).
19. Segal, D.M., Padlan, E.A., Cohen, G.H., Rudikoff, S., Potter,
    M. and Davies, D.R., Proc. Natl. Acad. Sci. U.S.A. 71:4298-4302
    (1974).
20. Edmundson, A.B., Ely, K.R., Girling, R.L., Abola, E.E.,

Schiffer, M., Westholm, F.A., Fausch, M.D. and Deutsch, H.F., Biochemistry 13:3816-3827 (1974).

21. Fehlhammer, H., Schiffer, M., Epp, O., Colman, P.M., Lattman, E.E. and Steigemann, W., Biophys. Struct. Mech. 1:139-146 (1975).

22. Wang, B.C., Yoo, C.S. and Sax, M., J. Mol. Biol. 129:657-674 (1979).

23. Kabat, E.A., "Structural Concepts in Immunology and Immunochemistry", 2nd Ed., Holt, Rinehart, and Winston, New York (1976).

24. Kabat, E.A., J. Immunol. 77:377-385 (1956).

25. Kabat, E.A., J. Cell. and Comp. Physiol. 50: suppl. 1:79-102 (1957).

26. Kabat, E.A., J. Immunol. 84:82-85 (1960).

27. Arakatsu, Y., Ashwell, G. and Kabat, E.A., J. Immunol. 97:858-866 (1966).

28. Cisar, J., Kabat, E.A., Dorner, M. and Liao, J., J. Exp. Med. 142:435-359 (1975).

29. Bhattacharjee, A.K., Das, M.K., Roy, A. and Glaudemans, C.P.J., Mol. Immunol. 18:277-280 (1981).

30. Schalch, W., Wright, J.K., Rodkey, S. and Braun, D.G., J. Exp. Med. 149:923-937 (1979).

31. Schepers, G., Blatt, Y., Himmelspach, K. and Pecht, I., Biochemistry 17:2239-2245 (1978).

32. Kranz, D.W. and Voss, E.W., Jr., Proc. Natl. Acad. Sci. 78:5807-5811 (1981).

33. Newman, B., Sugii, S., Kabat, E.A., Torii, M., Clevinger, B.L., Schilling, J., Davie, J.M. and Hood, L., (in preparation).

34. Bieth, J., Front. Matrix. Biol. 6:1-82 (1978).

35. Adams, J.M., Immunol. Today 1:10-17 (1980).

36. Honjo, T., Kataoka, T., Yaoita, Y., Shimizu, A., Takahashi, N., Yamawaki-Kataoka, Y., Nikaido, T., Nakai, S., Obata, M., Kawakami, T. and Nishida, Y., Cold Spring Harbor Symp. Quant. Biol. 45:913-923 (1981).

37. Kabat, E.A., Wu, T.T. and Bilofsky, H., "Sequences of immunoglobulin chains. Tabulation and analysis of amino acid sequences and precursor, V-regions, C-regions, J-chain, and β_2-microglobulin". Government Printing Office Publication NIH 80-2008, Washington, D.C. (1979).

38. Wu, T.T., Kabat, E.A. and Bilofsky, H., Proc. Natl. Acad. Sci. U.S.A. 73:617-619 (1976).

39. Klapper, D.G. and Capra, J.D., Ann. Immunol. (Inst. Pasteur) 127C:261-271 (1976).

40. Kabat, E.A., Wu, T.T. and Bilofsky, H., Proc. Natl. Acad. Sci. U.S.A. 75:2429-2433 (1978).

41. Milstein, C., Nature (Lond.) 216:330-332 (1967).

42. Kabat, E.A., Wu, T.T. and Bilofsky, H., J. Exp. Med. 152:72-84 (1980).

43. Tonegawa, S., Maxam, A.M., Tizard, R., Bernard, O. and Gilbert, W., Proc. Natl. Acad. Sci. U.S.A. 75:1485-1489 (1978).

44. Bernard, O., Hozumi, N. and Tonegawa, S., Cell 15:1133-1144 (1978).

45. Max, E.E., Seidman, J.G. and Leder, P., <u>Proc</u>. <u>Natl</u>. <u>Acad</u>. <u>Sci</u>. U.S.A. 76:3450-3454 (1979).
46. Sakano, H., Hüppi, K., Heinrich, G. and Tonegawa, S., <u>Nature</u> (Lond.) 280:288-294 (1979).
47. Weigert, M., Gatmaitan, L., Loh, E., Schilling, J. and Hood, L., <u>Nature</u> (Lond.) 276:785-790 (1978).
48. Early, P., Huang, H., Davis, M., Calame, K. and Hood, L., <u>Cell</u> 19:981-992 (1980).
49. Sakano, H., Maki, R., Kurosawa, Y., Roeder, W. and Tonegawa, S., <u>Nature</u> (Lond.) 286:676-683 (1980).
50. Komaromy, M. and Wall, R., <u>in</u>: "ICN-UCLA Symposia on Molecular and Cellular Biology", C. Janeway, E.E. Sercarz, and H. Wigzell, Vol. XX, p. 12, Alan R. Liss, Inc., New York (1981).
51. Sakano, H., Kurosawa, Y., Weigert, M. and Tonegawa, S., <u>Nature</u> (Lond.) 290:562-565 (1981).
52. Kurosawa, Y., von Boehmer, H., Haas, W., Sakano, H., Trauneker, A. and Tonegawa, S., <u>Nature</u> (Lond.) 290:565-570 (1981).
53. Kurosawa, Y. and Tonegawa, S., <u>J</u>. <u>Exp</u>. <u>Med</u>. 155:201-218 (1982).
54. Siebenlist, U., Ravetch, J.V., Korsmeyer, S., Waldmann, T. and Leder, P., <u>Nature</u> (Lond.) 294:631-635 (1981).
55. Wu, T.T. and Kabat, E.A., <u>Proc</u>. <u>Natl</u>. <u>Acad</u>. <u>Sci</u>. U.S.A. (in press).
56. Margolies, M.N., Cannon, L.E., Kindt, T.J. and Fraser, B., <u>J</u>. <u>Immunol</u>. 119:287-294 (1977).
57. Haber, E., Margolies, M.N., Cannon, L.E. and Rosemblatt, M.S., <u>Miami Winter Symp</u>. 9:303-338 (1975).
58. Matthyssens, G. and Rabbits, T.H., <u>Proc</u>. <u>Natl</u>. <u>Acad</u>. <u>Sci</u>. U.S.A. 77:6561-6565 (1980).
59. Wu, T.T., Kabat, E.A. and Bilofsky, H., <u>Proc</u>. <u>Natl</u>. <u>Acad</u>. <u>Sci</u>. U.S.A. 76:4617-4621 (1979).
60. Kabat, E.A., Wu, T.T. and Bilofsky, H., <u>J</u>. <u>Exp</u>. <u>Med</u>. 149:1299-1313 (1979).
61. Baltimore, D., <u>Cell</u> 24:592-594 (1981).
62. Egel, R., <u>Nature</u> (Lond.) 290:191-192 (1981).
63. Bothwell, A.L.M., Paskind, M., Reth, M., Imanishi-Kari, T., Rajewsky, K. and Baltimore, D., <u>Cell</u> 24:625-637 (1981).

NATURAL IMMUNITY AND MACROPHAGES

INTRODUCTORY REMARKS

M.L. Lohmann-Matthes

Max-Planck-Institut für Immunobiologie
D-7800 Freiburg, F.R.G.

15 years ago macrophage sessions, usually placed at the end of an immunology meeting, were apparently devoid of any interest to a real immunologist and were therefore at most occasions nearly empty except from the speakers and some discussants. In the meantime this picture has completely changed and "macrophages" have not only a full audience, but, as today, are happy to be put at the beginning of the meeting. What are the reasons for this development? If one looks at the contributions of today and takes also into account facts, which are not discussed today, one realizes that macrophages have successfully squeezed into most branches of immunological reactions. Although they have kept their nonspecific properties, they influence by various means specific immunological reactions. Some of the many secretory products of macrophages seem to be of high relevance for regulatory processes like Il-1 or prostaglandins. More directly macrophages influence immune reactions by presenting antigen associated to cell-membrane structures like Ia antigens. Whether or not this property is unique to macrophages or whether it is in fact also or exclusively a property of dendritic cells is still a matter of debate as well as the question, whether the dendritic cell is a cell type quite distinct from macrophages or whether these two cell types are related. Probably today these questions may be elucidated by the two presentations on dendritic cells and on macrophages both presenting antigen. Also in the area of natural killer cells, cells with macrophage surface antigens seem to play an important role as documented by several independent groups. However, also with these cells, which have in many respects the properties of T-cells there is no final evidence, whether they belong to the T-cell or to the macrophage lineage, whether they represent a cell line of their own, or whether they are precursor cells, which can be shifted into one or the other direction.

Finally, also in the area of cytotoxic reactions the macrophage plays an important role in the defense against tumor cells and micro-organisms. This cytotoxic property, however, is completely dependent on the activation by the T-cell lymphokine MAF and also probably on its counterpart MIF, which attracts macrophages to the site of an immune reaction. This broad variety of functions is one of the reasons, why macrophages are nowadays regarded as interesting part-ners in most immunological situations. One question, which will most probably be solved in the near future is, whether all the different functions are in fact performed by one cell type, which can acquire or lose functions according to its differentiation and maturation stage or whether also in the macrophage system functionally different subpopulations can be characterized.

ROLE OF MACROPHAGES IN T CELL ACTIVATION

P. Erb, G. Ramila, A. Stern, and I. Sklenar

Institute for Microbiology, University of Basel
Basel, Switzerland

INTRODUCTION

There is now general agreement that the induction of any immune
response is dependent on macrophages (MØ) or MØ-like cells which act
as antigen presenting cells. However, beside MØ, other cells which
are not considered to belong to the MØ lineage are also involved in
the induction of at least some immune processes. Thus, these
'inducer' cells are heterogeneous and the use of the term 'accessory
cells' (AC) or 'antigen presenting cells' (APC) instead of MØ seems
to be more appropriate to describe these cells. However, as a lot of
the evidence for antigen presentation has been obtained by studying
classical MØ, the term 'MØ' will be further used, keeping in mind
that the functional activities described will not necessarily be
restricted to this particular cell type.

Genetic restriction of MØ - T cell interactions

In 1973, Rosenthal and Shevach (1) showed that for antigen-
specific proliferation of guinea pig T cells MØ and T cells had to

---

Abbreviations:

AC: accessory cells; APC: antigen presenting cell; DC: dentric cells;
GRF: genetically related MØ factor; Ia: I region associated;
IAC: Ia-associated antigen complex; MHC: major histocompatibility
complex; MØ: macrophage(s); P cells: persisting cells, PEC: peritoneal exudate cells; Thc: T helper cells.

be identical at the major histocompatibility complex (MCH) in order
to cooperate successfully. This important observation was confirmed
by us in a different system, the induction of antigen-specific T
helper cells (Thc) in vitro (2,3). Thus, only MØ identical at the
I-A subregion of the H-2 complex induced or restimulated Thc. Since
then, the genetic restriction of T-MØ interactions in various systems has been firmly established (4-9).

Restriction means the involvement of I region products and it
was therefore obvious to look for Ia antigens on T cells and MØ.
While many attempts so far failed to demonstrate Ia antigens (coded
for by the I-A and/or I-E/C regions) on T cells, it was easy to
detect them on MØ (10-13). However, the various MØ populations differ in their expression of Ia antigen, eg. peritoneal exudate MØ
only contain a small proportion of Ia positive (Ia+) cells, while
the percentage of Ia+ monocytes or MØ in the spleen or thymus is
much higher. It is now clear that only Ia+ MØ express functional AC
activity. Thus, treatment of MØ with the appropriate anti-Ia sera
and complement abolishes their T cell activating property.

Regulation of Ia expression on MØ

Under in vitro culture conditions Ia+ splenic, thymic or peritoneal exudate MØ become Ia negative (Ia-) within a short time, ie.
one or two days (12,14,15). However, both synthesis as well as expression of Ia is resumed by these MØ provided they are exposed to
phagocytic stimuli such as bacteria, latex, zymosan, opsonized
erythrocytes, antigen-antibody complexes, or even antigen alone (15).
If these stimuli are added at the beginning of the culture period
they prevent the loss of the Ia expression for a prolonged time or
even enhance Ia expression (15). These in vitro results confirm in
vivo data, in which mice injected with Listeria, KLH or BCG showed
a marked increase of Ia+ MØ in the peritoneal exudate (16,17).

Beside phagocytic stimuli lymphokines obtained from ConA activated spleen cells (15), from Trypanosoma cruzi immune spleen
cells (18) or from Mycobacteria or Listeria immune T cells (19,20)
also enhance the synthesis and expression of Ia antigens on MØ in
vitro as well as in vivo demonstrating a T cell dependent regulation
of the synthesis and expression of Ia on MØ.

Thus, the expression of Ia on MØ is a transient event and it
correlates very well with the functional capacity of these MØ.

Accessory cell heterogeneity

As mentioned before, there is AC heterogeneity, ie. AC function
is not exclusively restricted to MØ or MØ-like cells. Other Ia+

cells such as dendritic cells (21), P cells (22) or some tumour lines of MØ or B cell origin (23,24) can also express AC activity for some T cell functions. The use of Ia+ tumour lines as AC is particularly useful, because as they represent a homogeneous (and sometimes even cloned) cell population, they may allow a much better insight into the mechanism of antigen presentation and T cell activation.

Thus, we tested whether tumour lines reported to induce T cell proliferation or T lymphokine production were also capable to function as AC for the activation of T helper cells. The tumour lines used were BC3A, a virus-induced leukemia, P388D1, a chemically induced MØ line and WEHI-3, an oil-induced myelomonocytic line. BC3A is Ia+, while P388D1 and WEHI-3 are Ia-, but Ia inducible by stimulation with certain lymphokines (eg. Con A Sup: supernatant from ConA activated spleen cells). As T cell functions antigen-specific T cell proliferation and helper activity for B cells were measured. A typical result is shown in Fig. 1. Starch-induced peritoneal exudate MØ (PEC) stimulate T cell proliferation as well as T cell help. BC3A and ConA Sup activated P388D1 only induce T cell proliferation but not T cell help. WEHI-3 (not stimulated with ConA Sup) neither induces T cell proliferation nor T cell help. The capacity of BC3A and P388D1 to function as AC in T cell proliferation was antigen-specific, MHC restricted and inhibitable by adding anti-Ia^d antibodies into the cultures. The results obtained demonstrate a fundamental difference between the activation of antigen-specific and Ia-restricted T cell proliferation and T cell help. This holds true for other tumour lines tested as well (data not shown). The reason for this difference is not yet known, but it is highly likely that it has something to do either with the uptake, processing or presentation of the antigen which might be different between normal MØ and transformed cells.

Mechanism of antigen presentation and T cell activation

Despite much efforts by many groups very little is known about the mechanism of antigen presentation and T cell activation at a molecular level. It is clear that MØ take up antigen, process it in a still unknown fashion and present it in context with Ia to T cells. T cell activation can be blocked at the level of the antigen presenting cell by appropriate anti-Ia antibodies but not by anti-antigen antibodies. This does not only suggest that Ia is involved in antigen presentation but also that the T cell receptor does not recognize antigen in its native form. This latter statement is also supported by the fact that adding an excess of soluble antigen into the cultures does not block T cell activation. Thus, the T cell receptor either recognizes the antigen in a modified form, eg. modified by the Ia and/or antigen processing, or the receptor will only become available for the antigen after prior interaction with Ia.

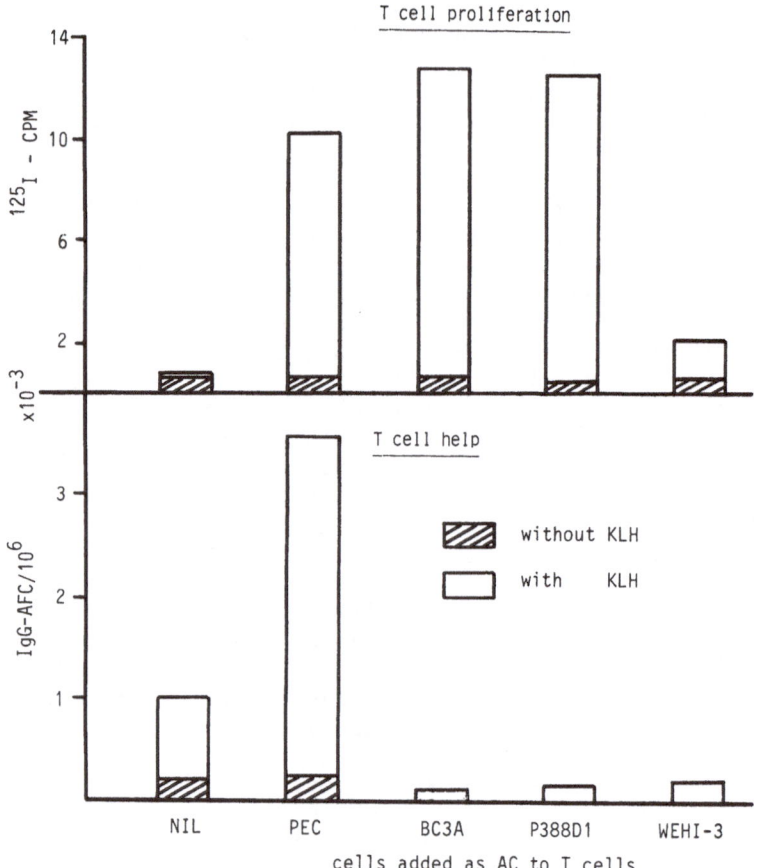

Fig. 1.   Highly purified lymph node T cells (purified by nylon wool
          and Sephadex G10 column filtration) obtained from KLH-primed
          BALB/c mice were incubated with or without KLH (10µg/ml) and
          with PEC, BC3A, P388D1 or WEHI-3, or without AC in microti-
          ter plates for 4 days. For T cell proliferation 3×10^5 T
          cells were incubated with 1×10^4 AC, for Thc activation 8×10^5
          T cells with 5×10^4 AC. To assess proliferation the uptake
          of ^{125}IUdR was measured which was added in a concentration
          of 0.25µc/well 8h before termination of the experiment. To
          assess helper activity, the cultures were harvested and
          5×10^4 viable cells added to 4×10^5 anti-Thy1 and complement
          treated DNP-primed BALB/c spleen cells and incubated to-
          gether with TNP-KLH (0.005µg/ml). After 5 days the IgG
          anti-DNP plaque response was measured (DNP and TNP cross-
          react at the antibody level) and calculated for 10^6 'B'
          cells.

Where to go from here? It is necessary to go in for that problem from two directions, from the T cell side as well as from the AC side. At the T cell level the nature of the receptor(s) recognizing antigen in context of Ia has to be revealed. By using T cell clones with defined antigen specificity in combination with the gene technology this task should be possible in due course. At the accessory cell level more information about the antigen presenting principle has to be found out. The study of the tumour lines, especially at a biochemical level will be very useful for that. Another way to look at that problem is the investigation of MØ factors which replace the AC function of MØ for T cell activation. Two such factors have been described, GRF (genetically related MØ factor) (25,26) and IAC (Ia antigen complex) (27). Both factors, although detected in quite different systems, express a striking similarity in terms of nature and functional property. Both consist of a complex of Ia antigen and immunogenic fragments which is formed as a consequence of the interaction of antigen with MØ. Both factors bind to and activate antigen-specific Thc in vitro as well as in vivo in a MHC restricted fashion and entirely replace the AC function of antigen-pulsed MØ or of MØ and antigen. The biochemical analysis of GRF or IAC (which is still very difficult to perform due to the minute amounts produced) should give us a lead about the antigen presenting principle and along with the information about the T cell receptor reveal the mechanism of T cell activation.

ACKNOWLEDGMENTS

This work was supported by the Swiss National Science Foundation (Grant Nr. 3:112-081) and the Juvenile Diabetes Foundation (Grant Nr. 80R058).

REFERENCES

1. Rosenthal, A.S. and Shevach, E.M., J. Exp. Med. 138:1194 (1973).
2. Erb, P. and Feldmann, M., Nature 254:352 (1975).
3. Erb, P. and Feldmann, M., J. Exp. Med. 142:460 (1975).
4. Miller, J.F.A.P., Vadas, M.A., Whitelaw, A. and Gamble, J., Proc. Natl. Acad. Sci. USA 72:5039 (1975).
5. Kappler, J.W. and Marrack, P.C., Nature 262:797 (1976).
6. Pierce, C.W., Kapp, J.A. and Benacerraf, B., J. Exp. Med. 144:371 (1976)
7. Thomas, D.W. and Shevach, E.M., J. Exp. Med. 144:1236 (1976).
8. Yano, A., Schwartz, R.H. and Paul, W.E., J. Exp. Med. 146:828 (1977).
9. Farr, A.G., Dorf, M.E. and Unanue, E.R., Proc. Natl. Acad. Sci. USA 74:3542 (1977).
10. Unanue, E.R., Dorf, M.E., David, C.S. and Benacerraf, B., Proc. Natl. Acad. Sci. USA 71:5014 (1974).

11. Schwartz, R.H., Dickler, H.B., Sachs, D.H. and Schwartz, B.D., Scand. J. Immunol. 5:731 (1976).
12. Cowing, C., Schwartz, B.D. and Dickler, H.B., J. Immunol. 120:378 (1978).
13. Stern, A.C., Erb, P. and Gisler, R.H., J. Immunol. 123:612 (1979).
14. Beller, D.I. and Unanue, E.R., J. Immunol. 124:1433 (1980).
15. Beller, D.I. and Unanue, E.R., J. Immunol. 126:263 (1981).
16. Beller, D.I., Kiely, J.M. and Unanue, E.R., J. Immunol. 124:1426 (1980).
17. Ezekowitz, A.B., Austyn, J., Stahl, P.D. and Gordon, S. J. Exp. Med. 154:60 (1981).
18. Steinman, R.M., Nogueira, N., Witmer, M.D., Tydings, J.D. and Mellman, I.S., J. Exp. Med. 152:1248 (1980).
19. Nussenzweig, M.C., Steinman, R.M., Gutchinov, B. and Cohn, Z.A., J. Exp. Med. 152:1070 (1980).
20. Scher, M.G., Beller, D.I. and Unanue, E.R., J. Exp. Med. 152:1684 (1980).
21. Steinman, R.M., Kaplan, G., Witmer, M. and Cohn, Z.A., J. Exp. Med. 149:1 (1979).
22. Schrader, J.W. and Nossal, G.J.V., Immunol. Rev. 53:61 (1980).
23. McKean, D.J., Infante, A.J., Nilson, A., Kimoto, M., Fathman, C.G., Walker, E. and Warner, N., J. Exp. Med. 154:1419 (1981).
24. Cohen, D.A. and Kaplan, A.M., J. Exp. Med. 154:1881 (1981).
25. Erb, P. and Feldmann, M., Eur. J. Immunol. 5:759 (1975).
26. Erb, P., Feldmann, M. and Hogg, N., Eur. J. Immunol. 6:365 (1976).
27. Puri, J. and Lonai, P., Eur. J. Immunol. 10:273 (1980).

ANTIGEN PRESENTATION BY DENDRITIC CELLS

Geoffrey H. Sunshine, Andrei A. Czitrom, Susan Edwards,
Marc Feldmann and David R. Katz

ICRF Tumour Immunology Unit, University College London
London, England

Until quite recently, the dogma on immune activation could be
summarized as follows: antigens were engulfed and devoured
(processed) by a specialized cell, the macrophage, characteristi-
cally adherent, phagocytic and radioresistant. A degraded fragment
of the consumed antigen then reappeared on the surface of the ingest-
ing cell and was then recognized by a T lymphocyte in association
with MHC subregion antigens (H-21 in the mouse) on this same
"fresser" cell (presentation) (1). Whilst it is clear that macrophages can certainly ingest and degrade antigens of all shapes and
sizes, there is little if any direct evidence that the events defined
by the term "presentation" are the responsibility of the same cell.
Thus, there is as yet no convincing evidence that antigen fragments
are actually re-expressed on the macrophage cell surface let alone
that they are presented or associated with macrophage H-21 antigens.

We therefore entertained the idea that other cells and other
mechanisms may be involved in antigen presentation. Our interest in
this area was kindled by the observations of Cowing and her colla-
borators who showed that when spleen adherent cells were pulsed with
antigen for 18 hours, the effective antigen presenting population was
now non-adherent whereas the adherent phagocytic macrophage population was almost totally ineffective (2). What was this non-adherent
antigen-presenting cell, a detached macrophage or a distinct cell
type? Support for the latter was provided by the seminal experiments
of Steinman and Cohn who had characterized a spleen cell with just
these properties (3). The cell was called "dendritic" because of its
characteristic appearance. It is now known to differ from the macrophage in a number of different physical traits and these are summarized in Table 1. Thus, the dendritic cell is nonphagocytic, lacks
Fc receptors (Fcr) and does not stain with the characteristic macro-

23

Table 1. Differences between dendritic cells and spleen macrophages
          (see refs. 3-6)

	Dendritic cells	Macrophages
Phagocytosis	−	+
Fc receptor	−	+
Adherence	+ → −	+ → +(+ → −)
Non-specific esterase	−	+
Appearance	Stellate, long processes	Rounded, blunt projections
Antigens		
I-A	+ → ±	+ → ±
mac-1, F4/80	−	+
33.D1	+	−

phage histochemical marker, non-specific esterase. I-A is expressed
on almost 100% of dendritic cells and at 5 to 7 times the level seen
on macrophages. Surface antigens also suggest fundamental differences
between macrophages and dendritic cells since the latter do not react
with two macrophage specific markers mac-1 and F4/80 whereas a new
monoclonal marker 33.D1 stains only dendritic cells (4).

In vitro function

     At the time of our first experiments, little was known of the
function of the dendritic cell except that it was described as a
potent stimulator of allogeneic (but not syngeneic or autologous)
T cell proliferation (5). We therefore isolated dendritic cells by
a modification of Steinman's density centrifugation method (6) and
asked if these purified cells would present exogenous, soluble antigen to purified T cells in a secondary proliferative response. A
typical experiment is shown in Table 2. Depleting primed lymph nodes
of endogenous presenting cells by adherence techniques substantially
depletes the antigen specific response. Similar results have also
been obtained by treating the lymph nodes with anti I-A plus complement (GHS, in preparation). Addition of GAT, the priming antigen, or

Table 2. Induction of antigen specific proliferation by different accessory cells

	96hr ^{125}IUdR incorporation***		
	0	50 µg/ml GAT	50 µg/ml PPD
Lymph Node*	2865	22.289	30.133
T cells**	1586	4.569	5.384
" + 5 x 10^3 2hr Ad cells	3025	16.347	20.149
" " Dendritic cells	3686	17.221	18.173
" " Spleen macrophage (AD.)	1798	2.066	2.954
" " " " (NAd.)	2034	3.087	4.129

* 2 x 10^5 draining lymph node cells from CBA mice primed with GAT in Complete Freund's Adjuvant 7 days earlier.

** 2 x 10^5 primed cells passed over nylon wool and Sephadix G10.

*** SD < 20% mean so omitted.

PPD, the antigen of Mycobacteria used in the adjuvant, in the presence of low numbers of irradiated syngeneic dendritic cells, resulted in almost complete restoration of the response. We have also seen dendritic cell presentation of other antigens such as keyhole limpet haemocyanin (KLH) and TGAL. Suprisingly, we also found that macrophages isolated at the same density as dendritic cells in these preparations were unable to reconstitute the depleted response.

These experiments raise further questions with profound implications for our thinking on antigen recognition by T cells. Is the non-phagocytic dendritic cell degrading antigen? If so is this occurring on the surface or at an intracellular site? Whilst antigens such as GAT and TGAL are reputed to be "sticky" and may attach to the surface membrane what does the dendritic cell do with an antigen the size of KLH (MW > 1x10^6)? These experiments do not formally prove that dendritic cells handle antigen and such proof has indeed been difficult to obtain subsequently. This may be due to technical problems (antigen dose, kinetics for example) or may suggest that perhaps another cell (an IA⁻ macrophage?) is involved. Similar considerations also apply in evaluating the antigen-presenting capabil-

ity of B cell lymphomas. These cells, presumably non-phagocytic and
I-A$^+$, also present soluble antigen to T cells in an almost indentical
system to that just described. Again, very low numbers induce antigen
specific proliferation but if antigen is pre-pulsed onto the B lymphomas almost one thousand-fold more cells are required to see significant T cell proliferation (7).

All these experiments challenge the primacy of the macrophage
as the putative antigen presenting cell and suggest that other cells
perhaps employing other pathways of antigen handling may also be involved. Do these experiments sound the death knell for the macrophage as antigen presenter? Although our experiments comparing macrophages and dendritic cells have been confirmed in rats using a mito-
genic system (8) it still seems too early to eliminate the macrophage: as originally indicated (6), we feel that other populations
of macrophages may well be active and based on the low recoveries
published for the rat it is possible that as yet untested macrophage
subpopulations may be active in that system. Furthermore, studies
using macrophages cloned from precursors in bone marrow strongly
suggest that at least some macrophages are effective (P.Erb, this
volume and 9).

We have also turned our attention to the original functional
observation with dendritic cells namely the stimulation of allogeneic
T cell responses. In this instance, it appears that the dendritic
cell presents not exogenous but endogenous surface antigens to the
allo T cell. Presentation of surface Ia is clearly important since
anti Ia sera block this response (10). In contrast with the original
observation we find, however, that splenic macrophages are also able
to activate both allo proliferation and cytotoxicity and this has
been confirmed by others (11,12). Since these same splenic macrophages were unable to activate GAT primed T cells, it would suggest
that the requirements for alloactivation are perhaps less stringent.
We originally suspected that this heterogeneity of stimulators might
have been due to individual stimulator populations activating distinct T cell subsets but we could find no evidence for this even
when cloned T cells were examined (in collaboration with A.
Glasebrook, A. Kelso and H.R. MacDonald, Lausanne). Table 3 illustrates one of the Ly1$^+$2$^-$ clones that was investigated: it responded
to low numbers of both dendritic cells and macrophages by prolif-
erating and secreting mediators (MAF and IL-2) (13). Other prolif-
erating Ly 1$^+$2$^-$ clones behaved similarly. What makes the dendritic
cell (or indeed the macrophage) such a potent stimulator of allogeneic responses remains to be clarified: one area we are now investigating is the cell's ability to make mediators such as IL-1
which may be involved in T cell triggering (14).

Table 3.   Induction of proliferation in clone AD5 (BALB/c anti
           DBA/2 = anti Mls[a])

| | T cell Response | | |
DBA/2 stimulator (2000R)	72 hr ^{3}H-TdR incorp	Production of: MAF	IL-2
10^6 spleen	+++	+++	+
2×10^4 dendritic cells	++	++	++
2×10^4 spleen macrophage	++	++	+

In vivo

We have also been intent on extending our in vitro findings to
in vivo antigen presentation. So far our data suggest that antigen
presenting cells are effective as stimulators in inducing cytotoxic
responses after injection into H-2 distinct mice, though it is not
clear whether dendritic cells are potent (AAC et al, in preparation).
Two systems have recently been described where dendritic cells may
be active in vivo. These are 1) rejection of long surviving kidney
grafts which have been depleted of passenger leucocytes-injection
of dendritic cells syngeneic to the graft causes rejection presumably by provoking an in vivo MLR (15) and 2) TNP-modified dendritic
cells when injected induce a form of contact sensitivity which is
hard to suppress in contrast to an easily suppressible or even suppressor form when modified macrophages are injected (16).

All these data taken together suggest that the physical differences between macrophages and dendritic cells reflect functional
differences between these important cell types. How the dendritic
cell works and how closely it is related to the macrophage are areas
which we feel will shed light on the complex question of immune
activation.

REFERENCES

1.   Rosenthal, A.S., Immunol. Rev. 40:136 (1978).
2.   Cowing, C. et al. J. Immunol. 121:1680 (1978).
3.   Steinman, R.M. and Cohn, Z.A., J. Exp. Med. 137:1142 (1973).
4.   Nussenzweig, M.C. and Steinman, R.M., Immunol. Today 3:65 (1982).
5.   Steinman, R.M. and Witmer, M.D., Proc. Nat. Acad. Sci. USA
     75:5132 (1978).

6. Sunshine, G.H., et al. J. Exp. Med. 152:1817 (1980).
7. Glimcher, L.H., et al. J. Exp. Med. 155:445 (1982).
8. Klinkert, W., et al. J. Exp. Med. 156:1 (1982).
9. Lee, K.C. and Wong, M., J. Immunol. 125:86 (1980).
10. Sunshine, G.H., et al. Eur. J. Immunol. 12:9 (1982).
11. Röllinghoff, M., et al. Eur. J. Immunol. 12:337 (1982).
12. Czitrom, A.A., et al. Immunol. 45:553 (1982).
13. Kelso, A., et al. J. Immunol. 129:550 (1982).
14. Durum, S.K. and Gershon, R.K., Proc. Nat. Acad. Sci. USA
    79:4747 (1982).
15. Lechler, R.I. and Batchelor, J.R., J. Exp. Med. 155:31 (1982).
16. Britz, J.S., et al. J. Exp. Med. 155:1344 (1982).

THE MACROPHAGE AS A CYTOTOXIC EFFECTOR CELL

IN MICE AND HUMANS

M.L. Lohmann-Matthes, H. Lang,
D. Krumwieh, and D. Sun

Max-Planck-Institut für Immunbiologie
D-7800 Freiburg, F.R.G.

INTRODUCTION

Activated macrophages are now generally agreed to be cytotoxic effector cells against tumor cells and intracellular microorganisms (1). The most potent activator is the lymphokine MCF (MAF) which apparently cooperates with or is enhanced by substances like LPS (2).

The most actual problems in research on macrophage cytotoxicity are the following: production of large quantities of the lymphokine (3-5) purification of MCF (6, 7), application of the in vitro puri- fied lymphokine in in vivo situations and most important the repro- ducibility of the mouse results with human cells. The present report focusses on the last two points.

MATERIALS AND METHODS

All methods used in the mouse system have been described else- where (8,9).

Production of human MCF (MAF)

a. Spleen cells were obtained from healthy donors after post- traumatic splenectomy. Erythrocytes were lysed and the mononuclear cells were activated for 48 h with 2γ Con A/ml in serum free medium (Dulbecco's modified Eagle's Medium, DMEM). b. Peripheral blood cells were passed through a one step Ficoll gradient. The interphase was plated for 30 min on surface treated plastic petri dishes to

remove most of the adherent monocytes. The nonadherent cells containing mostly lymphocytes and some monocytes (PBL) were stimulated for
48 h with 2γ Con A in serum free medium. The supernatants of both
types of cultures were used as MCF (MAF) containing lymphokine preparation.

Cytotoxic assay with human and mouse effector cells

To obtain human monocytes the Ficoll interphase of white peripheral blood cells was plated on surface treated petri dishes. After
30 min the nonadherent cells were removed by repeated washings and
the human monocytes were collected from the surface treated petri
dishes using a soft rubber policeman. These cells were then used
immediately as effector cells in flat bottomed microtiter plates.
Lymphokine preparations were added to the cells immediately as has
been described by Montovani et al. (10).

Human peritoneal cells were obtained from patients undergoing
chronical peritoneal dialysis and plated also first for 30 min on
surface treated petri dishes. The adherent cell population was then
transferred into microtiter plates. Human monocytes and peritoneal
cells were plated at a density of $2x10^5$ cells per well. To both populations MCF (MAF) containing lymphokine preparations were added
immediately. In the case of the monocytes also ^3H thymidine-labeled
TU_5 (10) cells were added on the same day and the assay was terminated 72 h later. In the case of the peritoneal cells target cells
were added on the second day according to the procedure used in the
mouse system and the assay was terminated 48 h later. The ratio
between effector cells and targets was 10:1. The percentage of ^3H
thymidine release into the supernatant was calculated according to
the formula:

$$\% \text{ cytotoxicity} = 100 \quad x \quad \frac{\text{cpm supernatant}}{\text{cpm sediment} + \text{cpm supernatant}}$$

All experiments were done at least 10 times in triplicate. The
data were highly reproducible. There was some variation in the
amount of spontaneous cytotoxicity of peripheral blood monocytes
from donor to donor. However, the increase by additional lymphokine
activations was very stable.

Mouse peritoneal cells were induced with thioglycollate and collected on day 4-6. They were immediately plated into microtiter
plates at a density of $1x10^5$ cells/well. They could be used as effector cells for up to one week. MCF was added for 24 h, than was
removed and labeled tumor target cells were added for another 24 h.

RESULTS

1. Macrophage cytotoxicity in the mouse

a. In vitro system. Mouse macrophages can be rendered cytotoxic by two different mechanisms, the antibody dependent mechanism and the lymphokine-induced mechanism. These two mechanisms differ in their lytic kinetics in as such, that the antibody-dependent cytotoxicity starts immediately after mixing of antibody, target cells and macrophages, whereas in the lymphokine system the macrophages need an activation period of about 18 h to become cytotoxic (11). As reported before these two mechanisms cooperate and enhance each other as documented in Figure 1 (11).

b. In vitro/in vivo systems. The next obvious step was to investigate, whether this macrophage cytotoxicity, working so reproducibly in vitro could be induced in vivo by injection of lymphokine preparations. Since we had in the meantime succeeded to separate MCF (MAF) from a variety of other lymphokines including MIF (6) we injected materials of different lymphokine activity intraperitoneally into mice. As documented in Table 1 MCF rich preparations induced strongly cytotoxic macrophages, whereas MIF rich preparations induced an increase in cell number without effect on cytotoxicity.

c. In vitro/in vivo experiments in tumor and infection models. The next approach was to inject MCF intraperitoneally, thus rendering

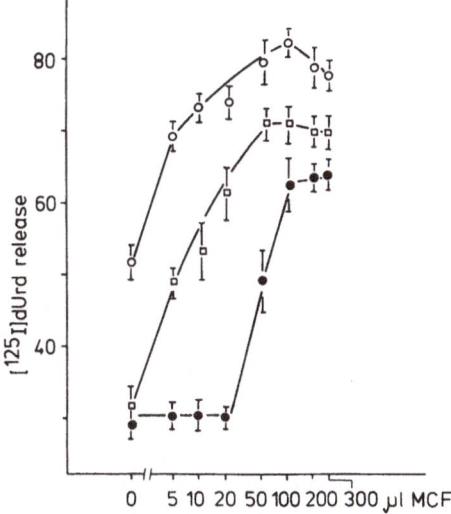

Fig. 1. Mouse macrophages can be rendered cytotoxic by two different mechanisms, the antibody dependent mechanism and the lymphokine-induced mechanism. These two mechanisms cooperate and enhance each other.

Table 1. Number and cytotoxicity of peritoneal macrophages of mice
          injected with different fractions of a lymphokine prepara-
          tion analyzed by isoelectric focussing.

Fraction from isoelectric focussing analysis injected i. p.	number of peritoneal macrophages	% spec. cytotoxicity P 815
Fraction pH 8,5 containing MCF	$9 \times 16^6 \pm 1$	31 ± 4
Fraction pH 5,5 containing MIF	$22 \times 10^6 \pm 2$	5 ± 1
Control fraction pH 11	$6 \times 10^6 \pm 1$	0 ± 4

The lymphokine preparation (ConA induced spleen cell supernatants)
was first passed through a Phenyl-Sepharose column and subsequently
applied to isoelectric focussing analysis in the presence of 4 m
urea (6). The eluted fractions were dialyzed overnight against phos-
phate buffered saline. C57BL/10 mice were injected 3 times.i.p.
within 36 h. 12 h after the last injection peritoneal cells were
collected and tested for cytotoxicity at an effector to target ratio
of 8:1 for 18 h.

the mouse macrophages cytotoxic and then exposing the mice to either
tumor cells or infectious agents. In the infection model we used
Salmonella typhimurium strain 1826 (kindly provided by Dr. Jann from
our institute). Table 2 demonstrates, that preactivation of the macrophages results in good protective effects against Salmonella typhimurium 1826.

In the tumor models we were less successful by the application
of MCF alone. Although a significant prolongation of survival was
obtained all animals died finally. Therefore, we applied the above
mentioned cooperative system and injected together with the tumor
cells syngeneic antiserum directed against the tumor cells. In all
experiments the animals which had received antiserum and MCF surviv-
ed completely, whereas antiserum alone had no effect and MCF only
a small one as mentioned above (Table 3). The experiments were done
with the BalbC Meth A tumor and with two freshly induced (Benzpyrene)
C57BL/10 fibrosarcomas kindly provided by Prof. Schmähl, Deutsches
Krebsforschungszentrum) (data not shown, Lang et al., in preparation).

Table 2. Protective effect of MCF (MAF) against an infection with
          Salmonella typhimurium SF 1826

Treatment of mice	Mean survival time (days) after the i.p. infection with Salmonella typhimurium SF 1826 infection dosis
PBS	10 fold LD_{50} 9 ± 1
MCF (MAF) 2 x 200 U/24 h	46 ± 5

C3H/f mice were injected at 12 h intervals i.p. with 200 U of MCF
(MAF). After 4 injections C3H/f mice were i.p. injected with
Salmonella typhimurium SF 1826. Treatment of mice with MCF (MAF)
was continued for 7 days.

Table 3. Influence of intraperitoneal application of MCF on tumor
          growth of Balb/c MethA cells

Pretreatment of Balb/c mice	i.p. tumor MethA inoculum	survival in days mean values of 10 animals
-	5×10^5	14
MCF (200 U)	5×10^5	19
-	5×10^5 coated with syngeneic anti-Meth A serum	18
MCF (200 U)	5×10^5 coated with syngeneic anti-Meth A serum	complete

Mice were injected i.p. with 200 U MCF at 12 h interval. The MCF
treatment was started 2 days before the inoculation of tumor cells
and was maintained for 7 further days.

2. Experiments using human lymphokines and effector cells

After many years of work in the mouse system we wanted to be sure, that the system works similarly also in the human situation. The preparation of the lymphokine was done according to the methods in the mouse. The test system however turned out to be exceedingly difficult to establish in a reliable and reproducible way.

a. Cytotoxicity test with human peripheral blood monocytes as effector cells. First we tested on human monocytes from the peripheral blood according to Montovani et al. (10). The data given here only figure out what we obtained with cells used directly on the day of isolation from the blood. In addition, we have done a careful time kinetic with cultured monocytes, which will be published elsewhere.

Table 4.   Cytotoxicity of untreated and in vitro lymphokine activated human monocytes tested against TU_5 cells

Effector cells	% release from ^3H thymidine labelled TU_5 cells
Spleen cell MCF incubated with human monocytes	50
PBL MCF incubated with human monocytes	49
Medium incubated with human monocytes	39
Medium alone without monocytes	20

Human monocytes were prepared as described in Materials and Methods. 2×10^5 monocytes were plated into each well of a 96-well-microtiter plate. Lymphokine preparations or medium were added together with labelled TU_5 cells. After 72 h the supernatants were collected and the released cpm counted in β counter. Ratio between monocytes and TU_5 cells was 10:1. TU_5 cells alone have a very low spontaneous isotope release. The presence of monocytes, which have not been stimulated, however, always shows a more or less pronounced spontaneous cytotoxicity, which can be, however, increased by additional lymphokine stimulation.

Table 5. Cytotoxicity of human peritoneal macrophages activated in
          vitro with human MCF and tested against mouse P815 tumor
          targets.

Effector cells	% ^{3}H thymidine release from prelabelled P815 cells
Peritoneal macrophages incubated 24 h with spleen MCF	55
Peritoneal macrophages incubated 24 h with PBL MCF	60
Peritoneal macrophages incubated 24 h with medium	25
Medium without peritoneal macrophages	26

Peritoneal macrophages were prepared as described in Material and
Methods. They were first incubated for 24 h with lymphokine preparations. Then ^{3}H thymidine labelled targets were added for 48 h at a
rate of 10 effector cells to 1 target.

The monocytes of a healthy donor are usually preactivated to a more
or less high degree so that the additional activation by lymphokines
is not very impressive (Table 4). This in vivo preactivation is apparently a sign of a perfectly well functioning lymphokine and macrophage system. However, because of these highly varying background
conditions this system is probably not suited for routine testing.

     b. Cytotoxicity test with human peritoneal cells. Cells were
obtained from 4 different donors every second day. These cells were
in most cases with one exception not preactivated and were therefore
beautiful effector cells in the lymphokine-dependent cytotoxicity
system. Table 5 shows, that with P815 mouse target cells using human
peritoneal macrophages as effector cells highly reproducible results
could be obtained, results comparable to those in the mouse system.

     It is very important to really test human MCF preparations on
human effector cells in order to avoid that during the chemical purification procedure one isolates a molecule from human origin which
activates only mouse but not human macrophages. Therefore, every new
step of purification has to be counter-checked with human effector
cells. For routine laboratory use, however, an animal test system

Table 6.   Cytotoxicity of mouse thioglycollate induced peritoneal
           macrophages activated with human MCF containing lymphokine
           preparations.

Effector cells	% ^{51}Cr release from P815 cells
Mouse PE macrophages activated 24 h with spleen MCF	70
Mouse PE macrophages activated 24 h with PBL	68
Mouse PE macrophages incubated 24 h with medium	30
Medium alone without PE macrophages	32

C57BL/10 mice from our conventional breeding colony, which are usually
exposed to a variety of inapparent infections were injected with 3 ml
thioglycollate solution i.p. on day 4 their peritoneal cells were
collected and plated at 1x10^5 cell/well in 96-well-microtiter plates.
The cells were then activated for 24 h. After this time the lymphokine was removed, the cells were washed and ^{51}Cr labelled P815 targets
were added at a ratio of 10:1. After 18-24h the assay was terminated.

offers many advantages.

    c. <u>Assay for human MCF on mouse peritoneal macrophages</u>. Therefore
we put a lot of effort on finding an appropriate mouse effector cell.
Resting peritoneal macrophages do not respond at all to human MCF
preparations, nor do bone marrow derived macrophages. However, thioglycollate macrophages of a slight degree of preactivation are ideal
effector cells even up to two weeks in culture. As shown in Table 6
these mouse thioglycollate-induced peritoneal cells respond in a
very sensitive and reproducible way to human MCF.

DISCUSSION

    The data presented with mouse material show, that <u>in vitro</u> pro-
duced MCF (MAF) is highly effective in activating <u>in vivo</u> peritoneal
macrophages. We have also tested Kupffer cells from the liver and
also these macrophages respond perfectly to MCF (data not shown).

The reported protective in vivo effects with Salmonella typhimurium 1826 must of course be pursued with microorganisms, which produce a slow progress of the infection, so that MCF can be applied after the onset of the infection. Also much better purified lymphokine preparations will have to be used in order to obtain a clearcut knowledge on MCF effects in vivo. However, these data are first hints, that in vitro produced MCF material is effective in vivo. In the case of the tumor experiments we failed to obtain good protective effects by the administration of MCF alone. Only the combination with antitumor antiserum gave convincing protective effects. Thus, one may speculate, that at least with the tumors used in our experiments only the combination of MCF and antitumor antiserum works in the tumor situation. Many tumors, however, are known to produce circulating antibodies like e.g. melanomas. Such tumors may thus be ideally suited for treatment with MCF. Along this line Fidler has reported good effects of MCF (MAF) treatment melanoma B16 in mice (12).

For a long time we had great problems to establish a reliable and reproducible test system for human MCF. With the described techniques we are now in the lucky position to be able to test human MCF both with human and mouse effector cells and both human and mouse targets. From our data it is quite clear that there is no species specificity for MCF at least not in the direction human/mouse.

For the future of course we shall focus on the further purification of MCF by use of affinity chromatography with monoclonal anti-MCF antibodies and on the further in vivo use of this purified material.

REFERENCES

1. Lymphokine reports No. 3. E. Pick and M. Landy ed. in: "Macrophage activation", Academic Press (1981).
2. Hibbs, J.B., Taintor, R.R., Chapman, H.A. and Weinberg, J.B., Science 197:279 (1977).
3. Sun, D., Krumwieh, D. and Lohmann-Matthes, M.L., Immunobiology 160:120 (1981).
4. Schreiber, R.D., Altman, A. and Katz, D.H., J. Exp. Med. 156:677 (1982).
5. Ratliff, T.L., Thomasson, D.L., McCool, R.E. and Catalona, W.J., Cell. Immunol. 68:31 (1982).
6. Kniep, E.M., Domzig, W., Lohmann-Matthes, M.L. and Kickhöfen, B., J. Immunol. 127:417 (1981).
7. Leonard, E.J., Ruco, L.P. and Meltzer, M.S., Cell. Immunol. 41:341 (1978).
8. Lohmann-Matthes, M.L., Lang, H., Sun, D., Kniep, E.M. and Kickhöfen, B., in: "Lymphokines", E. Pick and M. Landy, eds. Vol. 3, p. 365, Academic Press (1981).
9. Meerpohl, H.G., Lohmann-Matthes, M.L. and Fischer, H., Eur. J.

      Immunol. 6:213 (1976).
10. Montovani, A., Jerrelis, T.R., Deau, J.H. and Herberman, R.B.,
      Int. J. Cancer 23:18 (1979).
11. Lang, H. and Lohmann-Matthes, M.L., Immunobiology 157:109 (1980).
12. Fidler, J.J., Science 208:1469 (1980).

A CELL-FREE PRODUCT SECRETED BY LY⁻2⁺ CELLS CAN INDUCE

A MOLECULE REQUIRED FOR LY2 SUPPRESSOR CELL ACTIVITY

Patrick M. Flood, Diane Louie, and Richard K. Gershon

Department of Pathology
The Howard Hughes Institute for Cellular Immunology
Yale University School of Medicine
New Haven, Connecticut 06510, U.S.A.

INTRODUCTION

The generation of suppression to SRBC in vitro involves the interaction of different T cell subsets in a well defined regulatory "feedback" circuit. The cells of this circuit have been identified by the correlation of function with a unique profile of cell surface glycoproteins (differentiation antigens). The induction signal is delivered by an I-J⁺ Ly1⁺2⁻ cell to an Ly1⁺2⁺ I-J⁺ acceptor cell (1,2). The interaction between the Ly1 inducer cell and the Ly1,2 transducer cell is antigen-specific and restricted by genes linked to the V-region of the immunoglobulin heavy chain locus. The transducer cell then activates the effector cell of the suppressor circuit. One mechanism by which this takes place is the differentiation of transducer cells into effector cells (3). Other mechanisms may exist. The effector cell is so called because of its ability to suppress Ly1 cells directly, without the need for an Ly1,2 transducer cell (4). These effector cells are capable of suppressing not only helper cells, but also the feedback inducer cells. This results not only in a shutdown of antibody synthesis but abrogates additional T suppressor induction and thereby completing the feedback circuit. The phenotype of the effector cell is an Ly1⁻2⁺ and, unlike the other cells of the feedback circuit, it does not bear the I-J subregion gene products (4). This is especially important in light of the fact that the interaction between the suppressor effector cell and its target is partially restricted by genes mapping into this same I-J subregion of the MHC.

Cell free products secreted by cells of the suppressor circuit which functionally mimic T suppressor inducer cells (Ly1 TsiF) or

T suppressor effector cells (Ly2 TsF) have facilitated the analysis
of cellular interactions in the suppressor circuit. The Ly1 TsiF
consists of two molecules, one of which binds antigen and the other
which bares I-J, has no antigen specificity, and is the source of
the Igh-V linked genetic restriction of the inducer factor (5).
Recent evidence suggests that each molecule is produced by a different cell (or the same cell in different stages of differentiation)
(6). The biochemical relationship of these two molecules and the
mechanisms by which they act in consort to successfully induce the
suppressor feedback circuit are currently under investigation, but
current evidence suggests no genetic or physical interaction exists
between the two chains (unpublished observations).

    The action of Ly2 TsF is quite different. Ly2 TsF consists of
one chain (or two chains covalently linked) which bears no MHC region
markers, but acts in an MHC-restricted manner to directly suppress
Ly1 cells. Recent evidence suggests that although Ly2 TsF is produced
by the suppressor effector cell, this effector cell is not the terminal cell of the suppressor circuit. Elimination of Ly1 I-J$^+$ cells
from the assay population, while not affecting the PFC response of
the B cells, completely abrogates the ability of Ly2 TsF to suppress
that response (7). The requirement for the I-J$^+$ cell can be circum-
vented by adding a molecule secreted by Ly1 T cells. This I-J$^+$ molecule can come from the I-J$^+$ fraction of Ly1 TsiF, or can be induced
in vitro by Ly2 TsF from 48 hr cultures of Ly1 cells (8). Thus, the
I-J$^+$ fraction of the Ly1 TsiF contains two activities. One is involved in the induction signal for suppression and acts upon transducer cells. The other cooperates with the Ly2 TsF to act upon helper
T cells (in the absence of suppressor transducer cells). We asked
whether these activities were the property of a single molecule or
two separate molecules.

    The second activity can be directly induced by the action of
the Ly2 TsF on I-J$^+$, Ly1 T cells in the helper cell assay population.
We report here experiments in which the dynamics of this interaction
were investigated. This induced I-J$^+$ molecule was then examined for
its ability to replace the I-J$^+$ molecule in the signal for suppressor
induction. We found that successful induction of the I-J$^+$ molecule
by Ly2 TsF requires both specific antigen and MHC homology between
the Ly2 TsF and the cells secreting the material. Further, this material is I-J$^+$, antigen non-specific, and does not replace the I-J$^+$
molecule needed for suppressor induction. Therefore, the Ly2 TsF can
function as a one chain suppressor molecule only in so far as it can
induce the production of a "partner" molecule, a molecule which
works in tandem with the Ly2 TsF to effect suppression on the Ly1$^+$
T helper cell.

MATERIALS AND METHODS

Mice: C57BL/6, Balb/c, B10.D2 and C57BL/10J mice, 6-10 weeks of age, were obtained from Jackson Laboratory, Bar Harbor, Maine. Balb. B, Balb.K, C.B20, B.C9, and Bab. 14 were bred at Yale University School of Medicine.

Antisera: Monoclonal anti-Ly sera were generously supplied by F.W. Shen, Memorial Sloan-Kettering Cancer Center, New York. Monoclonal anti-Thy-1 reagents were generously provided by Dr. Jonathan Sprent, University of Pennsylvania, Philadelphia, P.A. Anti-I-J[b] serum was prepared by hyperimmunizing B10.A(5R) recipients with a mixture of B10.A(3R) spleen and lymph node cells (antiserum No. ASM-20). Anti-I-J[k] was prepared by hyperimmunizing B10.A(3R) recipients with a mixture of B10.A(5R) spleen and lymph node cells (antiserum ASM-18). (We thank D.B. Murphy for preparing these antisera). Depletion of cells bearing Lyt or I-J markers was achieved by incubating 1×10^7 cells/ml of antibody appropriately diluted in balanced salt solution (BSS) (1:1000 for anti-Ly monoclonal antibody, 1:5 for anti-Thy-1 monoclonal antibody hybridoma supernatant, or 1:5 for anti-I-J serum), washing, and incubating with complement for 45 minutes at 37°C (1×10^7 cells/ml of rabbit serum diluted 1:10 for anti Ly or anti-I-J antibody or 1×10^7 cells/ml of guinea pig complement for anti-Thy-1 antibody). Complement used in these experiments was serum from animals selected for low natural cytotoxicity to mouse spleen cells.

Antigens: Sheep erythrocytes (SRBC) were obtained from Colorado Serum Company Laboratories, Denver, Colorado.

Method of Cell Preparation: Spleen cells were washed in BSS and suspended in RPM1 1640 supplemented with antibiotics, 10% fetal calf serum (FCS), 100mM glutamine, 25mM Hepes, and 5×10^{-5}M 2-mercaptoethanol for tissue culture. T cells were prepared by adding unprimed spleen cells to plastic petri dishes coated with goat anti-mouse immunoglobulin and harvesting the nonadherent fraction(s) (9). B cells were prepared by treating the cells with monoclonal anti-Thy-1 and complement.

Preparation of Lyt 1⁺ derived suppressor inducer (Lyl TsiF) and Lyt 2⁺ derived suppressor effector (Ly2 TsF) materials: Preparation of Lyl TsiF and Ly2 has been previously described (1,2). Briefly, a suspension of spleen cells from mice hyperimmunized with SRBC was treated with anti-Lyt 2(for Lyl TsiF) or anti-Lyt 1 (for Ly2 TsF) and rabbit complement, and subsequently cultivated in vitro for 48 hrs in RPMI 1640 + 10% FCS at a concentration of 10^7 cells/ml. After 48 hrs, supernatant fluids were cleared and passed through millipore filters.

Absorption of soluble factors: Absorption with erythrocytes was done by mixing 1 ml of culture supernates with 0.1 ml of a 50% suspension of sheep erythrocytes for 1 hr on ice. The erythrocytes were removed by centrifugation. For absorption with anti-I-J sera, supernatant fluids were passed over an anti-I-J immunosorbent (ASM-20) prepared by conjugation of antisera to cyanogen bromide-activated Sepharose.

Primary cultures: Lyl T cells at 10^7 cells/ml were incubated for 48 hrs with antigen (SRBC) and Ly2 TsF added at a final dilution of 1:5. Supernatants were then cleared, then passed through a millipore filter.

Assay cultures: Suppressor activity of the Lyl TsiF or the Ly2 TsF was determined by adding these materials to cultures of unprimed spleen cells that had been treated with various test reagents. All cells were suspended in culture medium, at a concentration of $2x10^6$ T cells and $2x10^6$ B cells in 1 ml, and cultured with 0.05ml of a 1% SRBC suspension in Falcon 3008 plates (Falcon Labware, Div. of Becton, Dickinson and Co., Oxnard, CA) in a 5% CO_2 - 95% air incubator at 37°C. The number of plaque forming cells (PFC) were determined on day 5 by using the Cunningham modification of the Jerne-Nordin plaque assay as previously described (10). Results are given as the mean of 3 individual calculations from each culture condition.

Isolation of I-J$^+$ molecule: Supernatants containing Lyl TsiF or from primary Lyl T cell cultures, were passed over the appropriate immunosorbant column made from anti-I-J antisera coupled to Sepharose 4B. After extensive washing, the column was eluted with 0.2M sodium carbonate (Na_2CO_3)pH 11.0. The eluted material was concentrated to original volume, and dialyzed overnight against first PBS, then RPMI 1640.

RESULTS

An Lyl I-J$^+$ cell needed for Ly2 TsF activity can be replaced by a molecule induced in primary culture by Ly2 TsF: Previous results have shown that the action of Ly2 TsF can be abrogated by treatment of splenic T cells with anti-Ly2 and anti-I-J (7). Suppressor activity can be returned to Ly2 TsF by addition of an I-J$^+$ molecule found in Lyl TsiF. We investigated whether the role of the Lyl I-J$^+$ cell needed for Ly2 TsF activity was to provide this I-J$^+$ molecule, and whether this cell can be activated to secrete its product by the action of Ly2 TsF. In order to test this hypothesis, spleen cells were depleted of Ig$^+$ cells and treated with anti-Ly2 antibody and complement, then incubated for 48 hrs with antigen and Ly2 TsF. The supernatant from these cultures were then tested for their ability to replace the need for the I-J$^+$ cell in the Ly2 TsF mediated suppression (Table 1). While Ly2 TsF can suppress Lyl T cells directly (lines 1+2) it can no longer suppress Lyl T cells depleted of I-J$^+$

Table 1. Ly2 TsF induces an activity in supernatants of Ly1 T cell cultures which overcomes the need for I-J$^+$ cells in the assay culture

Ly2 TsF in 1° culture[a]	B6 cells in assay culture	Ly2 TsF in 2° culture	% suppression of PFC response to SRBC	Comments
-	Ly1 T+B	-	standard	
-	Ly1 T+B	B6	70	Ly2 TsF suppresses Ly1 cells directly
B6	Ly1 T+B	-	60	
B6	Ly1 T+B	B6	75	Supernatant from Ly2 TsF activated 1° culture does not affect Ly2 TsF-mediated suppression when Ly1 I-J$^+$ cell present
-	Ly1 I-J⁻T+B	-	standard	
-	Ly1 I-J⁻T+B	B6	10	anti-I-J treatment does not affect PFC response / Ly2 TsF can no longer suppress
B6	Ly1 I-J⁻T+B	-	5	
B6	Ly1 I-J⁻T+B	B6	65	Ly2 TsF plus supernatant from Ly2 TsF-activated 1° cultures replaces need for J$^+$ cell

[a]1° culture consisted of Ly2 TsF at 1:10 with 10^7 unprimed B6 Ly1$^+$, 2$^-$ T cells for 48 hrs. For details see materials and methods.

cells (lines 5+6). Supernatant from primary cultures of Ly1 T cells
was able to replace the need for the I-J$^+$ cell, but only if the primary culture contained Ly2 TsF (lines 7+8). Removal of an I-J$^+$ cell
from the primary culture eliminated the ability of Ly2 TsF to induce
this activity in the supernatant (data not shown). It seems, therefore, that the Ly2 TsF can induce the production of a molecule which
functionally substitutes for an Ly1 I-J$^+$ cell. Further, this induction is not only dependent on the presence of an Ly1 I-J$^+$ cell, but
also requires antigen in the primary culture (unpublished observations).

Molecule which replaces the need for an Ly1 I-J$^+$ cell in the
assay culture is I-J$^+$ and antigen nonspecific: Primary supernatants
which replace the I-J$^+$ cell in Ly2 TsF mediated suppression were
passed over an anti-I-J immunosorbant to determine if the molecule
induced by the Ly2 TsF is I-J$^+$ (Table 2). While Ly2 TsF in secondary
culture failed to suppress the response of Ly1 I-J$^-$ T+B (lines 1+2),
addition of primary supernatant induced with Ly2 TsF replace suppressive activity (line 3). Supernatant passed over an anti-I-Jb immunosorbant shows that the "I-J replacing" molecule in the supernatant
contains the I-J^b haplotype marker (lines 4+5). Passage of the same
supernatant over an anti-I-J^k immunosorbant resulted in no activity
being retained in the column (lines 6+7). In addition, absorption of
supernatant with the antigen used to induce the I-J$^+$ chain reveals
that this molecule does not bind antigen (line 8).

Induction of the I-J$^+$ molecule by Ly2 TsF requires homology at
MHC between Ly2 TsF and target cells: We investigated the genetic
restrictions involved in the induction of the I-J$^+$ molecule by Ly2
TsF (Table 3). Ly2 TsF from B6, Balb/c, and congenics at both the
Igh and H-2 gene loci were used to induce the I-J$^+$ molecule in primary culture. The results show that only Ly2 TsF from H-2 compatible
mice can induce the I-J$^+$ material. Ly2 TsF from animals which match
B6 at Igh but not H-2 were unable to induce the I-J$^+$ molecule from
Ly1 cells. Two important groups must be noted here: while Balb/c
Ly2 TsF was unable to induce I-J$^+$ material from B6 cells factor from
its H-2^b congenic partner Balb.B was as good as syngeneic factor
at inducing this material; conversely, B6 Ly2 TsF was able to induce
the I-J$^+$ molecule while B10.D2 was not. The results from these two
strains clearly indicate that MHC homology between Ly2 TsF and the
cells in the primary culture is essential if these cells are to be
induced to secrete I-J$^+$ material.

The I-J$^+$ molecule induced by Ly2 TsF cannot functionally replace
the I-J$^+$ molecule in Ly1 TsiF: Since previous results have shown
that a I-J$^+$ molecule from Ly1 TsiF could mimic the functional activity of the I-J$^+$ molecule induced by Ly2 TsF (7), we tested if the
converse was also true, i.e. if the Ly2 TsF induced I-J$^+$ molecule
could mimic the I-J$^+$ molecule needed for Ly1 TsiF activity
(Table 4). Ly1 TsiF was fractionated into antigen-binding chain and

Table 2. Active molecule induced by Ly2 T_sF in 1° culture is
I-J^{b+} and antigen non-specific

Ly2 T_sF in 1° culture[a]	treatment of supernatant from 1° culture	B6 Ly2 T_sF in 2° culture	% suppression of PFC response to SRBC
–	–	–	standard
–	–	B6	0
B6	–	B6	85
B6	I-J^b Filtrate	B6	15
B6	I-J^b Eluate	B6	70
B6	I-J^k Filtrate	B6	75
B6	I-J^k Eluate	B6	0
B6	SRBC absorbed	B6	70

[a]See footnote a, Table 1
[b]Assay culture consisted of 2×10^6 Ly1$^+$, 2$^-$ I-J$^-$ cells = 2×10^6
 B cells from B6 mice. For details see materials and methods.

I-J$^+$ chain by passage over an anti-I-J immunosorbant, and this I-J$^+$
molecule was added to either Ly1 TsiF antigen-binding chain or Ly2
TsF to test for the ability to reconstitute suppressor activity.
Likewise, I-J$^+$ material induced in primary culture by syngeneic Ly2
TsF, was used to reconstitute Ly1 or Ly2 TsF activity. Ly1 TsiF activity was measured on whole T+B cultures, while Ly2 TsF activity
was measured on Ly1 I-J$^-$ T+B cultures. The results show that I-J$^+$
material from either Ly1 TsiF or Ly2 TsF induced cultures can restore Ly2 TsF activity (lines 7-9) but only I-J$^+$ material from Ly1
TsiF could restore the suppressive activity of Ly1 TsiF antigen-
binding chain. Therefore, it appears that while Ly1 TsiF contains
I-J$^+$ material which has more than one specificity, the I-J$^+$ material
induced by Ly2 TsF can only work in consort with Ly2 TsF for suppressive activity, and does not contain the specificity which is
needed to functionally replace the I-J$^+$ material normally needed
for the induction of suppression by Ly1 TsiF.

DISCUSSION

    In earlier studies we described an antigen-specific suppressor
factor (Ly1 TsiF) which required the action of two separate macromolecules to deliver its inductive signal (5). One molecule gave

Table 3. Induction of I-J$^+$ molecule by Ly2 T$_s$F is MHC restricted

Ly2 T$_s$F in 1° culture[a]	Identity of Ly2 T$_s$F with cells in 1° culture		Ly2 T$_s$F in Assay Culture	% suppression of PFC response to SRBC[b]
	H-2	Igh		
—			—	standard
—			B6	0
B6	+	+	B6	70
BC-9	+	—	B6	65
CB20	—	+	B6	0
Balb/c	—	—	B6	0
Balb.B	+	—	B6	55
B10	+	+	B6	75
B10.D2	—	+	B6	10

[a] See footnote a, Table 1
[b] See footnote b, Table 2

the factor antigen specificity and comes from a cell which is I-J$^-$ the other gives the factor a V$_H$ restriction and comes from a cell which is I-J$^+$. Recently we discovered a similar situation with other antigen-specific suppressor factor: Ly2 TsF. Although this molecule appears to require only one molecule for suppressive activity, further investigation revealed that this molecule carries with it the ability to induce the production of a "partner" molecule by cells in the assay population. Removal of this cell renders the Ly2 TsF incapable of effecting suppression. So, like Ly1 TsiF, the active, suppressive molecular complex of Ly2 TsF consists of two molecules, one which is antigen binding, the other of which is I-J$^+$ and is the source of the Igh-V linked genetic restriction.

In the current set of experiments, we attempted to dissect the series of interactions involved in the production of a functionally active hybrid molecule with the ability to suppress Ly1 T helper cells directly. We learned that: a) Ly2 TsF plus the relevant antigen were capable of inducing an I-J$^+$ molecule which overcame the need for an Ly1 I-J$^+$ cell in the assay culture: b) the induction of this molecule was MHC restricted: and c) the molecule was exquisitly specific in the suppressor circuit for Ly2 TsF. It therefore appears that while the Ly2 TsF has potent suppressor activity, it also has the ability to induce a cell activity as well, depending

Table 4. I-J$^+$ molecule induced by Ly2 T$_s$F does not replace Ly1 T$_{si}$F activity

Source of J$^+$ material[a]	Source of antigen-specific molecule	% suppression of PFC response to SRBC		Comments
		whole T+B	Ly1$^+$, 2$^-$I-J$^-$T+B	
Ly1 T$_{si}$F	—	standard	standard	I-J$^+$ molecules alone do not suppress PFC responses of either culture
Ly2 T$_s$ F induced	—	0	0	
	—	15	15	
—	Ly2 T$_s$F	55	0	Ly2 T$_s$F can suppress whole T, but not Ly1 cells depleted of J$^+$ cells.
Ly1 T$_{si}$F	Ly2 T$_s$F	60	55	J$^+$ molecule from Ly1 T$_{si}$F or induced by Ly2 T$_s$ F can restore suppressive activity.
Ly2 T$_s^-$ F induced	Ly2 T$_s$F	70	70	
—	Ly1 T$_{si}$F	15	ND[b]	Ag binding chain of Ly1 T$_{si}$F alone does not suppress.
Ly1 T$_{si}$F	Ly1 T$_{si}$F	65	ND[b]	J$^+$ chain from Ly1 T$_{si}$F but not Ly2 T$_s$F induced can replace suppressive activity.
Ly2 T$_s$F induced	Ly1 T$_{si}$F	15	DD[b]	

[a] J$^+$ material was either isolated from Ly1 T$_{si}$F as described, or was made from Ly1 cell cultures induced by Ly2 T$_s$F (see footnote a, Table 1).

[b] not done

on which cell is targeted by this factor. Although it remains to be
determined if it is the same molecule which induces I-J$^+$ chain production that later works in tandem with it to effect suppression, a
novel mechanism may be at work here: a single molecular entity may
have both an inducing and suppressing activity depending upon the
target cell. The first molecule induces its "schlepper" (carrier)
chain, then this "schlepper" chain carries this molecule to its appropriate target cell, which is then turned off by this molecular
suppressor complex.

How might this mechanism work? There are of course a number of
different hypothesis which may explain this data, but we would like
to put forth one that seems most intriguing. First, the functional
Ly2 TsF must recognize its intermediary cell through some specific
interaction mechanism. We have already found that in order for Ly2
TsF to successfully interact with the I-J$^+$ molecule, they must both
be a product of cells which share I-J polymorphisms. Therefore, one
can envision that the binding of Ly2 TsF to antigen may cause the
exposure of a receptor on the Ly2 TsF which can specifically recognize the I-J$^+$ molecule on the membrane of the intermediary cell. The
interaction of the Ly2 TsF with the membrane bound I-J$^+$ receptor molecule can activate the cell via a transmembrane signal, much the
same way many hormones do (for review, see ref. 11). Once activated,
the cell begins to secrete I-J$^+$ molecules which form a functionally
active hybrid molecule. The functionally active molecular complex is
then targeted onto its target cell via an antigen bridge, and the
schlepper molecule signals the target cell to internalize the functionally suppressive antigen binding chain. This signal between the
I-J$^+$ chain and the target cell receptor is Igh-V linked. This places
the H-F restriction of the Ly2 TsF on the induction and interaction
with the I-J$^+$ molecule, and the subsequent Igh-V restriction on the
interaction of the schlepper molecule with its target cell.

The reason we assign functional suppressor activity to the antigen binding chain is twofold: a) Fresno and colleagues (12,13)
have shown a clonal T suppressor factor with antigen binding activity to have functional suppressor activity; and b) one can make an
artifical suppressor factor using antigen binding Ly2 TsF and choleratoxin B chain as the schlepper molecule. This molecule will
supress any cell with a receptor for choleratoxin B chain. Therefore, we have replaced the active A chain of choleratoxin with our
own suppressor factor and have achieved suppressive activity. For
these reasons, we feel quite confident in assigning suppressive activity to the antigen-binding and not the I-J$^+$ chain of the active
suppressor complex.

The question is now raised whether this scheme can be used as a
general model for other antigen-specific T suppressor molecules. So
far we have found at least three molecular complexes in the suppressor circuit which require two separate macromolecules, one of which

is an I-J$^+$ schlepper chain, to deliver the biologically active signal (5,7,14). Other workers also report similar findings (15,16). The important generalization we wish to make from these studies are that of a two chain model in which one acts as a schlepper chain to focus the functional molecule on the appropriate cell receptor so that the functional molecule may enter the cell and perform its function inside the cell. In this model, some functional molecules may have the ability to induce their own schlepper molecules, but absolutely require this schlepper molecule for effecting its designed function.

To sum up, we describe here a molecular complex with six active sites: a) the antigen-binding specificity of the Ly2 TsF, which imparts the antigen restriction to the factor; b) the anti-I-J receptor on the Ly2 TsF, which imparts a genetic restriction on the interaction of Ly2 TsF and the I-J$^+$ molecule; c) the inducing sight on Ly2 TsF for the I-J$^+$ molecule, which may or may not be related to the anti-I-J receptor; d) the I-J$^+$ determinant on the schlepper molecule; e) the Igh-V linked restricting element on the schlepper molecule; and f) the suppressive moiety on the Ly2 antigen-binding TsF. These six sites must work in consort to form an antigen-specific suppressor effector molecule.

REFERENCES

1. Cantor, H. and Gershon, R.K., Fed. Proc. 38:2058 (1979).
2. Yamauchi, K., Murphy, D.B., Cantor, H. and Gershon, R.K., Eur. J. Immunol. 11:905 (1981).
3. McDougal, J.S., Shen, F.W., Cort, S.P. and Bard, J., J. Immunol. 125:1157 (1980).
4. Yamauchi, K., Murphy, D.B., Cantor, H. and Gershon, R.K., Eur. J. Immunol. 11:913 (1981).
5. Yamauchi, K., Chao, N., Murphy, D.B. and Gershon, R.K., J. Exp. Med. 155:655 (1981).
6. Chao, N., Thesis, Yale University School of Medicine, New Haven, Connecticut (1981).
7. Flood, P.M., Yamauchi, K. and Gershon, R.K., J. Exp. Med. 156:361 (1982).
8. Flood, P.M. and Gershon, R.K., manuscript in preparation.
9. Wysocki, L.J. and Sato, V.L., Proc. Natl. Acad. Sci. U.S.A. 75:2844 (1978).
10. Cunningham, A.J. and Szenberg, A., Immunology 14:599 (1968).
11. Catt, K.J. and Dufau, M.L., in: "Endocrinology and Metabolism", P.H. Felig, J.D. Baxter, A.H. Broadus, and L.A. Frohman, Eds., pp. 61-105 (1981).
12. Fresno, M., McVay-Boudreau, L., Furthmayr, H. and Cantor, H., J. Exp. Med. 153:1246 (1981).
13. Fresno, M., McVay-Boudreau, L., Nobel, G. and Cantor, H., J. Exp. Med. 153:1260 (1981).

14. Ptak, W., Rosenstein, R.W. and Gershon, R.K., Proc. Natl. Acad. Sci. U.S.A. 79:2375 (1981).
15. Taniguchi, M., Saito, T., Tahei, I. and Tokuhisa, T., J. Exp. Med. 153:1672 (1981).
16. Taussig, M.J. and Holliman, A., Nature (Lond.) 277:308 (1979).

FREQUENCY-ANALYSIS OF PRECURSORS OF CYTOTOXIC T LYMPHOCYTES IN
RADIATION CHIMERAS: ENUMERATION OF ANTIGENSPECIFIC CTL-P
RESTRICTED TO THYMIC MHC- AND BONE MARROW-MHC-DETERMINANTS

Klaus Pfizenmaier, Hubertus Stockinger, Martin Krönke,
Peter Scheurich, Conny Hardt, Martin Röllinghoff and
Hermann Wagner

Institut für Med. Mikrobiologie, Universität Mainz
6500 Mainz, Augustusplatz, FRG

INTRODUCTION

The mechanisms controlling the acquisition of T cell restriction specificity and immunocompetence are, despite of numerous investigations, not well understood. From studies of the CTL-immune
responsiveness in thymus- and bone marrow-grafted chimeric mice,
it became apparent, that it is the thymus which is crucial not only
for the maturation or T cells, but also for the specificity repertoire of the T cells (1,2). From these data it was suggested, that
during intra-thymic maturation both mutational events and positive
selection mechanisms influence the repertoire such that only T
cells restricted to thymic epithelial cell MHC determinants mature
and will be exported to the peripheral lymphoid organs (3,4). However, the demonstration of non-thymic MHC restricted CTL in both
chimeric (5-7) as well as conventional mice (8-10) are incompatible
with models proposing strictly thymus-dependent selection mechanisms. Allo-MHC restricted T cells were found not only within spleen
cells, but also within thymocytes of both chimeric (9) and non-
chimeric mice (10). Accordingly, both self- and allo-MHC restricted
thymocytes mature to immunocompetent T cells.

In previous studies the influence of the thymus for the T cell
restriction specificity has been approached by analyzing cytotoxic
or proliferative T cell responses either in vivo (1,8,11) or in
vitro in mass-mixed lymphocyte cultures (2,4-7). Due to the contro-
versial data obtained, it became necessary to further evaluate the
existence and the quantitative relationship of self-versus allo-MHC
restricted T cells. We have therefore used the limiting dilution

technique (12,13) to enumerate precursors of virus- and hapten-
specific cytotoxic T cells in thymus- and bone marrow grafted chimeric mice. In a first series of experiments, where we have investigated the Sendai-virus specific immune response in fully allogeneic
chimeras we found comparable frequencies of thymus and bone marrow-
MHC restricted CTL-P, irrespective of the MHC-type of the thymus-
graft (14,15,16). We also noted in most mice higher frequencies of
bone marrow-restricted CTL-P, and only in some mice a thymic MHC
preference of CTL-P. We have continued these studies and will here
present data on Sendai-virus and TNP-specific CTL-P which, in summary, suggest that the restriction phenotype of peripheral cytotoxic T cell precursors is not strictly dictated by the thymic MHC
type, that is, maturation of CTL-P can occur independent of their
restriction specificity.

RESULTS AND DISCUSSION

     From our earlier results (14), where we have found higher fre-
quencies of bone marrow restricted Sendai virus-specific CTL-P in
fully allogeneic chimeras, the question was raised to which extent
environmental priming could have resulted postthymically in a preferential expansion of bone marrow MHC-restricted clones due to a
lack of appropriate antigen-presenting cells for the thymic MHC restricted CTL-P population. To approach this question, chimeras were
constructed from adult thymectomized (CBA x BALB)F_1 $|(P_1 x P_2)F_1|$
mice, grafted with parental (P_1 or P_2) neonatal thymus prior to
lethal irradiation (900 R) and subsequent reconstitution with anti-
theta-treated parental (P_1 or P_2) bone marrow cells in four different combinations Pl/Pl, P_2/P_1, P_2/P_2 as described (14). We have
compared the CTL-P frequencies within spleen cells of such chimeras
which had been either left untreated (not intentionally primed) or
were primed intraperitoneally with Sendai-virus 2 weeks prior to in
vitro limiting dilution analysis. A representative example of the
data obtained, where the CTL-P frequencies of individual chimeras
are listed, is given in Table 1. The data reveal, that in all non-
primed mice, the frequency of H-2^d restricted Sendai-virus specific
CTL-P was around 1/ 35 000 (range 1/15 000 1/55 000) and the H-2^k restricted CTL-P were found with a frequency of 1/25 000 (range
1/12 000-1/54 000). Thus, irrespective of the combination of thymus
and bone marrow the same order of magnitude of H-2^d restricted and
H-2^k restricted CTL-P existed in spleen cells of chimeric mice.
However, if one compares, in individual mice, the frequencies of
H-2^d restricted with H-2^k restricted CTL-P, preferences become apparent; for example Pl/P2 reconstituted mice contained greater
numbers of self-MHC-restricted compared to allo-MHC-restricted CTL-P
(Table 1, no. 1,5). This finding closely parallels the situation
found in both spleen cells and thymocytes of unmanipulated mice.
Here, upon removal of allo-reactive T cells, by in vitro negative
selection procedures, self- and allo-MHC- restricted virus specific

Table 1. Sendai-virus specific CTL-P frequencies in spleen cells of chimeric mice:
Preferential expansion of self-restricted CTL-P due to priming

Chimera: (CBA x BALB/c)F$_1$ host

| No. | origin of | | in vivo | frequency of Sendai-virus specific CTL-P restricted | |
	bone marrow	thymus	priming	BALB/c (H-2^d)	CBA (H-2^k)
1	BALB/c	BALB/c	no	1/ 31 000	1/54 000
2	BALB/c	BALB/c	yes	1/ 8 000	1/30 000
3	BALB/c	CBA	no	1/ 39 000	1/12 000
4	BALB/c	CBA	yes	1/ 4 000	1/ 9 000
5	CBA	CBA	no	1/ 55 000	1/16 000
6	CBA	CBA	yes	1/200 000	1/ 3 000
7	CBA	BALB/c	no	1/ 15 000	1/16 000
8	CBA	BALB/c	yes	1/ 32 000	1/ 6 000

CTL-P can be demonstrated, the self-MHC restricted CTL-P being in a
3-5 fold excess over allo-MHC-restricted CTL-P (9,10). The question,
whether this self preference reflects thymus dependent selection
mechanisms was approached by the analysis of H-2-incompatible chimeras of the type P_1/P_2 and P_2/P_1 using F_1 animals as a host for the
bone marrow and thymus graft (Table 1, no. 3,7). Indeed, in individual mice we did find higher frequencies of thymic MHC-restricted
CTL-P compared to bone marrow restricted CTL-P (Table 1, no. 3); in
other mice, no clear preference could be demonstrated (Table 1,
no. 7). Although these data can be interpreted in terms of intrathymic selection of T cells' restriction phenotype, they clearly con-
tradict models proposing a strict positive selection and concomitant
maturation of thymus MHC restricted T cells only (3,4). In contrast
to the latter assumption is also the demonstration of bone marrow-MHC
restricted virus specific cytotoxic T cells within an allogeneic
thymus, where it is apparent that these CTL-P have indeed matured
intrathymically (9). We have here shown that bone marrow restricted
CTL-P may be found in peripheral lymphoid organs with frequencies
not too much different from thymic MHC-restricted CTL-P (Table 1).
This led us to argue that intrathymic acquisition of immunocompetence
of CTL-P has to be separated from mechanisms qualitatively and quantitatively influencing the specificity repertoire of T cells.

In contrast to the frequency values determined in unprimed chimeras of the P_1/P_2 type, primed chimeras of the same type contained
higher frequencies of CTL-P restricted to the MHC type of the bone
marrow, while the number of thymic-MHC-restricted CTL-P remained
roughly the same as under non-primed conditions (Table 1, no. 4,8).
For example, in spleen cells of the allogeneic chimera no. 3, a 3
fold excess of thymus-MHC restricted CTL-P was determined and in a
chimera of the same type (no. 4), but primed with Sendai virus previously, the ratio of thymus-to bone marrow-restricted CTL-P was
found to be 1 to 2. Similarly, the excess of self-MHC restricted
CTL-P observed in chimeras of the P_1/P_1 and P_2/P_2 type, is more
pronounced upon priming. This finding was not unexpected despite the
fact that the host animal is of F_1 origin. The chimeras have been
immunized 6-8 months after reconstitution, and one can assume that
during this time period the lymphoreticular system (LRS) of the host
has been largely replaced by bone marrow derived cells from the parental donor (17). As stimulation of T cells requires cells of the
LRS, priming will result in a selective expansion of self- (i.e.
bone-marrow) restricted CTL-P. The reasoning that postthymic expansion of CTL-P selectively occurs for self-MHC restricted CTL-P as
a consequence of priming, may account for the variation of Sendai-
virus specific CTL-P frequencies in earlier chimera studies (14).

We have, therefore, in a next series of experiments investigated the CTL-immune response of chimeras against the hapten TNP,
where it is less likely that environmental priming influences the
quantitative composition of the peripheral T cell pool.

The chimeras were used 2–3 months after reconstitution. They were constructed as described above using as a host (CBA x B6)F_1 animals which had been reconstituted with B6 or CBA thymi and B6 or (CBA x B6)F_1 bone marrow cells. Spleen cells of these chimeras were stimulated for 6 days in mass cultures (3 x 10^6 responder, 2 x 10^6 TNP conjugated cells) of CBA or B6 origin stimulator in the presence of 10% Interleukin-2 containing culture supernatants. The data given in Table 2 evidenced that all types of chimeras studied were able to generate TNP specific CTL. The restriction phenotype of the CTL-population induced apparently was dependent on the H-2 type of the stimulator cell employed. H-2 typing of the effector cells of mouse no. 3 and 4 (Table 2) revealed, that both $H-2^b$ and $H-2^k$ restricted CTL-activity was abolished by anti-$H-2^b$ and not by anti-$H-2^k$ and complement treatment, indicating the B6 origin of the effector cells, whereas CTL-activity of the F_1 cell reconstituted mouse no. 1 and 2 was abrogated by both anti-$H-2^b$ and anti-$H-2^k$ treatment of effector cells (data not shown). It is interesting to note, that irrespective of the type of chimera used we found a preferential $H-2^k$ restricted TNP specific CTL response. This haplo-type preference is apparently similar to that described for non-chimeric mice of the $H-2^k$ and $H-2^b$ haplotype (18,19). On the basis of the data presented here it is tempting to speculate that the observed haplotype preference resides primarily on the level of the antigen presenting cells. In addition, it appears that the thymic environment in which T cells differentiate influence this preferential responsiveness on the T cell level. The data in Table 2 illustrate this reasoning: the B6/B6 chimera (no. 4) is a better responder towards the allogeneic CBA-TNP-stimulator cells compared to the syngeneic B6-TNP stimulator cells. As in the F_1/B_6 chimera (no. 1) we find here in terms of lytic units roughly a 5 fold $H-2^k$ -preference. It is obvious, that this preference cannot be a result of intrathymic positive selection mechanisms. However, it may be a reflection of the different antigenicity of TNP conjugated $H-2^k$ versus TNP conjugated $H-2^b$ cells. The arguments for an additonal haplotype preference on the level of T cells stem from the observation that both B6 and Fl bone marrow cells, differentiating in a chimera grafted with a CBA thymus, have an even more pronounced $H-2^k$ response, which again is about five-fold better than in mice grafted with a B6 thymus. These findings suggest that under the influence of an $H-2^k$ thymus the T cells' specificity repertoire is further bended towards $H-2^k$ restriction.

We have then asked whether the thymus' influence on restriction phenotype of TNP specific CTL-immune-responses, as seen in bulk cultures (Table 2), is manifested on the level of the cytotoxic precursor cell, or on regulatory cells. We have therefore performed a limiting dilution analysis to estimate the TNP specific CTL-P frequency. These experiments were done with a different batch of chimeras than the experiments described in Table 2. The chimeric mice were constructed from (CBA x B6)F_1 hosts and from (CBA x BALB/c)F_1 hosts, which were thymectomized and reconstituted with parental type thymi

Table 2. Induction of TNP-specific, thymus- and bone marrow restricted CTL in spleen cells of chimeric mice

Chimera: (CBA x B6)F$_1$ host

No.	origin of bone marrow	origin of thymus	treatment of effector cells[†]	stimulator cells CBA-TNP target cells CBA 30:1	CBA-TNP 30:1	CBA-TNP 6:1[††]	C57-TNP target cells C57 30:1	C57-TNP 30:1	C57-TNP 6:1
1	F$_1$	B6	–	-3	51	39	2	34	21
2	F$_1$	CBA	–	5	60	45	0	26	10
			–	9	50	40	5	19	17
3	B6	CBA	α–b	–	6	5	–	0	0
			α–k	–	45	40	–	22	13
			–	0	36	17	4	22	14
4	B6	B6	α–b	–	3	4	–	3	2
			α–k	–	28	17	–	18	10

† MLC-cells were harvested 6 days after stimulation with TNP conjugated spleen cells and incubated with either rabbit complement alone (–), or with anti H-2^b (1/40) allo-antiserum (α–b) or with a monoclonal anti H-2^k antibody (1/1 000) (α–k), followed by complement treatment. Cells were washed twice and tested for cytotoxic activity against ^{51}Cr-labelled ConA-lymphoblasts in a 4 hours assay.

†† Effector to target cell ratio.

and bone marrow. Spleen cells of these chimeras were analysed 6 months after reconstitution for frequencies of TNP specific CTL-P. The data summarized in Table 3 confirm our studies on the Sendai-virus specific CTL-P frequencies (Table 1). The TNP specific frequencies were again in the same order of magnitude for both MHC-types involved. We also noted a slightly greater number of thymus-restricted CTL-P in 3 out of 4 of the allogeneic chimeras tested. However, it remains open, whether the observed differences indicate intrathymic positive selection or just reflect the variation found among individual mice of the same type (for example no. 3 and 5). The average frequency for $H-2^k$ restricted CTL-P of 3 out of 4 chimeras was 1/20 000 (exp. 1, no. 2,3) and the $H-2^b$ restricted CTL-P frequency was in all 4 chimeras 1/30 000. Essentially similar data were obtained in the second experiment listed in Table 3, where chimeras of the CBA/BALB/c combination were investigated.

With respect to the preferential $H-2^k$ restricted responsiveness of chimeric spleen cells in mass culture, the data obtained in the subsequently performed frequency analysis were surprising. Thus, we found very similar numbers of both $H-2^k$ and $H-2^b$ restricted TNP specific CTL-P (Table 3, exp. 1). The minor differences in frequencies of $H-2^k$ versus $H-2^b$ restricted TNP specific CTL-P are unlikely to account for the profound difference in the generation of CTL in mass cultures (Table 3). This is particularly true if one considers that the frequency of $H-2^k$ restricted CTL-P in chimeras grafted with B6 (no. 1) or CBA thymi (no. 2,3) were virtually the same. Because the data presented in Table 2 (mass culture) and Table 3 (limiting dilution) were obtained in independent experiments, we cannot yet conclude whether or not the CTL-P frequency is the critical parameter for H-2 preference in TNP specific responses. Nevertheless, the data are compatible with the view that the H-2 preference seen in bulk cultures is on one hand a matter of antigen presentation and on the other hand controlled by thymus dependent regulatory (helper ?) cells, and does not primarily reside at the level of CTL-P.

In conclusion, the analysis of the splenic CTL-P frequency for Sendai-virus and TNP in various thymus and bone marrow reconstituted chimeric mice has clearly established the existence of both self- and allo-MHC restricted CTL-P, irrespective of the MHC-type of the thymic graft. Similar data have been recently reported by Kruisbeek et al.: both host- and thymus-restricted TNP specific CTL were generated with spleen cells of nude mice engrafted with semi-allogeneic or fully-allogeneic thymi (20). In contrast, using thymocytes of the same animals as responders, only thymus-restricted CTL were induced. It was therefore concluded that, in nude mice, there exist both intra- and extra-thymic differentiation pathways of T cells, which apparently differ with respect to mechanisms selecting the restriction phenotype of T cells (20). This finding, however, contrasts our previous demonstration of allo-MHC restricted thymocytes in un-

Table 3. TNP specific CTL-P frequencies in spleen cells of chimeric mice

Chimera			origin of		Precursor frequency		
Exp.	No.	host	bone marrow	thymus	CBA-TNP	B6-TNP	BALB/c TNP
1	1	(CBAxB6)F$_1$	B6	B6	1/18 000	1/28 500	-
	2		CBA	CBA	1/21 000	1/34 000	-
	3		B6	CBA	1/17 500	1/28 000	-
	4		B6	CBA	1/65 000	1/30 000	-
2	1	(CBAxBALB/c)F$_1$	BALB/c	BALB/c	1/62 000	-	1/70 000
	2		CBA	CBA	1/17 000	-	1/28 000
	3		CBA	BALB/c	1/40 000	-	1/27 000

manipulated mice: after negative selection of alloreactive precursor cells, the ratio of TNP-specific CTL-P restricted to allogeneic versus self-MHC determinants ranged from 1/10 to 1/3 (10).

We have further shown, that within thymocytes of $(P_1 \times P_2)F_1$ chimeras, grafted with P_1 thymus and P_2 bone marrow, both P_1 and P_2 restricted CTL-P were present (9). A possible explanation for the lack of host-restricted thymocytes in the experiments of Kruisbeek et al. might be that the thymus grafted nude mice were tested early (1 month) after reconstitution (20) whereas we have used the allogeneic radiation chimeras 3 months after reconstitution (9). If indeed, as suggested by Longo and Schwartz (21), a bone marrow derived components of the thymus rather than thymic epithelial cells influence the restriction phenotype of maturing T cells, the reconstitution time becomes a critical parameter in the analysis of the development of T cells restriction specificity.

ACKNOWLEDGEMENTS

This work was supported by the Sonderforschungsbereich 107 and the Stiftung Volkswagenwerk.

The skilled technical assistance of Sabine Barth, Ute Münzing, Beate Maxeiner and Dagmar Tessmann is gratefully acknowledged.

REFERENCES

1. Zinkernagel, R.M., Callahan, G.N., Klein, J. and Dennert, G., Nature (London) 271:251-253 (1978).
2. Bevan, M.J. and Fink, P.J., Immunol. Rev. 42:4-19 (1978).
3. Zinkernagel, R.M. and Doherty, P.J., Adv. Immunol. 27:51-177 (1979).
4. von Boehmer, H., Haas, W. and Jerne, N.K., Proc. Natl. Acad. Sci. USA 75:2439-2441 (1978).
5. Matzinger, P. and Mirkwood, G., J. Exp. Med. 148:84-92 (1978).
6. Hünig, T. and Schimpl, A., Eur. J. Immunol. 9:730-736 (1979).
7. Wagner, H., Röllinghoff, M., Rodt, H. and Thierfelder, S., Eur. J. Immunol. 10:521-525 (1980).
8. Doherty, P.C. and Bennink, J.R., J. Exp. Med. 150:1187-1194 (1979).
9. Stockinger, H., Pfizenmaier, K., Hardt, C., Rodt, H., Röllinghoff, M. and Wagner, H., Proc. Natl. Acad. Sci. USA 77:7390-7394 (1980).
10. Stockinger, H., Bartlett, R., Pfizenmaier, K., Röllinghoff, M and Wagner, H., J. Exp. Med. 153:1629-1639 (1981).
11. Zinkernagel, R.M., Callahan, G.N., Althage, A., Cooper, S., Klein, P.A. and Klein, J., J. Exp. Med. 147:882-896 (1978).
12. Taswell, C., MacDonald, H.R. and Cerottini, J.C.,

Thymus 1:119–128 (1979).

13. Miller, R.G., Teh, T.S., Harley, E. and Phillips, R.A., Immunol. Rev. 35:38–58 (1977).

14. Wagner, H., Hardt, C., Bartlett, R., Stockinger, H., Röllinghoff, M. and Pfizenmaier, K., J. Exp. Med. 153:1517–1532 (1981).

15. Wagner, H., Hardt, C., Stockinger, H., Pfizenmaier, K., Bartlett, R. and Röllinghoff, M., Immunol. Rev. 58:95–129 (1981).

16. Wagner, H., Hardt, C., Heeg, K., Pfizenmaier, K., Solbach, W., Bartlett, R., Stockinger, H. and Röllinghoff, M., Immunol. Rev. 51:215–256 (1980).

17. Zinkernagel, R.M., Callahan, G.N., Althage, A., Cooper, S., Streilein, J.W. and Klein, J., J. Exp. Med. 147:897–911 (1978).

18. Levy, R.B. and Shearer, G.M., J. Exp. Med. 149:1379–1392 (1979).

19. Shearer, G.M., Schmitt-Verhulst, A.M., Pettinelli, C.B., Miller, M.W. and Gilheany, P.E., J. Exp. Med. 149:1407–1423 (1979).

20. Kruisbeek, M., Sharrow, S.O., Mathieson, B.J. and Singer, A., J. Immunol. 127:2168–2176 (1981).

21. Longo, D.L. and Schwartz, R.H., Nature (London), 287:44–46 (1980).

NEW LOCI IN HLA

J.J. van Rood, A. van Leeuwen and A. Termijtelen

Department of Immunohaematology and Blood Bank
University Hospital, 2333 AA Leiden
The Netherlands

The present paper deals with new (i.e. newly defined) loci recognized in the HLA complex: (1) we will outline the general approach
which in our experience has been the most successful for identifying
reagents for new loci, (2) we will discuss the recently recognized
class II locus SB/PL3 and (3) we will discuss a new class I locus
(or maybe better: class IV locus), TCA, possibly located within HLA
as well.

(1) The identification of reagents for new loci. If one
wants to identify a new locus, all one has to do is to select unrelated individuals which are identical or compatible for the established HLA antigens. Cellular reagents which may recognize new determinants, can then be raised in primed lymphocyte testing (PLT)
or cell mediated lympholysis (CML) techniques. Similarly, antibodies
recognizing non-HLA-A, -B, -C or -D/DR structures can be identified
by testing sera on a panel of lymphocytes which are HLA compatible
or identical with the serum producers. We call this the HLA-CAP
(compatible with antibody producer) approach. Although we are here
not physically capping the HLA-A, -B, -C and -DR antigens, in the
protocol used we have as little interference from them as when they
were capped. This approach has been exemplified in Table 1. This
table shows the reaction patterns of a selection of sera obtained
from 115 multiparous, HLA-A1-B8 and -DR3 positive women. These sera
were screened against lymphocytes from 9 different HLA-A1-B8-DR3
homozygous donors, implying that each positive reaction was directed
against a "new" determinant. The analysis of these reaction patterns
will be discussed later.

(2) The SB/PL3 locus. In Table 2 it is shown how the cellular
equivalent of the HLA-CAP approach can be used in PLT. Responder

61

Table 1.   Anti-monocyte antibodies found in sera from parous
           women with one HLA-Al-B8-DR3 haplotype

Donor[x] SB

```
BER  1,4   + + + + + + + + + + + + - - - - - - - - -
EYS  1,4   - - - + + + + + + + + + + + + + + - - - - -
HOV  4     - - - - - + + + + + - - - + + - - + + + - -
HAR  4     - - - - - + + + + + + + - + - + + - - - - +
POU  1     - - - - - - - - - + - - - - - - - - - - + +
HAG  1,2   - - - + - - - - - + + + + - - - - - - - + +
OVE  ND    - - - - - - - - - - - - - - - - - - - - -
JAN  2     - - - - - - - - - + + + - - + + + - - - - +
GYS  1,3   - - - - - - - - - + - - - - - - - - - - + +
```

ND = not done; x = all donors of the lymphocyte panel were
HLA-Al-B8-DR3 homozygous.

lymphocytes were sensitized towards HLA-D/DR compatible stimulator
lymphocytes. These PLT cells specifically recognized a determinant
(designated PL3A) which was associated with HLA-Al, -B8 and -Dw/DR3
but was different from any of these antigens. Individuals were found
which were positive for PL3A but negative for HLA-Al, -B8 and -Dw/DR3
and vise versa. This is an indication that the PL3A determinant is
governed by a locus separate from HLA-A, -B and -DR. It was found
to segregate with HLA in 3 informative families and with the B-D
end of the haplotype in an HLA-A, HLA-B recombinant (1). The existence of two additional alleles of PL3A, i.e. PL3B and PL3C, was
postulated on the basis of reactivity patterns in primary MLC in a
group of eleven Dw3 homozygous cells (2).

In 1980 Shaw et al. (3) also by raising PLT cells between
HLA-D/DR identical individuals, identified an HLA linked polymorphic
system of alloantigens. This so called secondary B cell or SB system was shown to carry at least 5 alleles (SB1 to 5). In a collaborative study with Shaw we were able to type a panel for SB1 to 5. PL3A
was found to be identical to SB1, PL3B turned out to give a complete
fit with SB4. Moreover, SB1 was shown to be identical to a determinant previously described by Mawas et al. (4) who generated PLT
cells between HLA identical siblings which differed for this determinant due to a recombination. Recently the SB/PL3 locus has been
mapped between HLA-D/DR and GLO1 (5).

Our panel which had been typed for SB1 to 5 included 18 homozygous typing cells (HTCs) obtained from the offspring of first
cousin marriages. Such cells are selected to be homozygous for HLA-A,

Table 2.   PL3A, a new determinant defined by PLT

PLT responder: Dw3, Dw8 (PL3A⁻)
PLT stimulator: Dw3, Dw3 (PL3A⁺)

Group 1	Group 2	++	+–	–+	––
PL3A	HLA-A1	10	3	19	57
PL3A	HLA-B8	8	5	19	57
PL3A	HLA-Dw/DR3	8	5	19	57

-B and -D/DR, but the question was whether they would also be homozygous for the SB determinants. Our finding was that 15 out of
18 HTCs carried only one SB determinant (i.e. were most likely homozygous for SB) but 3 HTCs carried two different SB alleles (Table 3).
An extension of these studies to the families of the donors confirmed
that the PL3/SB locus is situated between HLA-D/DR and GLO1, possibly as much as 2 cM away from the HLA-D/DR locus (manuscript in
preparation).

The first evidence that the SB determinants are carried by class
II molecules came from immunochemical studies with the monoclonal
antibody ILR1 (6). This antibody which is reactive with lymphocytes
from donors which are positive for SB2, SB3 or DR5 (7), preticipates
a glycoprotein composed of 2 polypeptide chains (MW = 29 000 and
34 000 daltons).

We were interested to see whether we would be able to identify
allo-antisera which contain antibodies recognizing the alleles of
the SB system. Over a thousand platelet absorbed sera were screened,
using the tests for the identification of B-cell antibodies, but no
good SB reagents were found. Next we decided to use the HLA-CAP approach. Over 100 sera obtained from HLA-A1-B8-DR3 positive women
which produced strong leucocyte antibodies, were tested against lymphocyte suspensions obtained from HLA-A1-B8-DR3 homozygous individuals. The two colour fluorescence (TCF) technique was used, which
allows the recognition of antibodies against B cells, T cells and
monocytes independently, without the need to separate these
cells (8). In this technique which is a complement dependent cytotoxicity test, ethidium bromide was used as a dye for dead cells,
which is a more sensitive reagent to test for viability than the
eosine stain normally used. We could identify 22 sera which reacted
with non-HLA-A, -B, -D/DR determinants. Positive reactions were
either found with monocytes alone or with monocytes and B-cells.
It turned out that the reaction pattern of 4 of these sera showed
a good fit with SB4, whereas the reaction pattern of one serum correlated with SB1+4. Next these 5 sera were absorbed with buffycoat

Table 3.   HLA-D/DR, SB and GLO1 phenotypes of 18 HTCs
           obtained from the offspring of first cousin
           marriages

Cell identification	HLA-D	HLA-DR	SB	GLO1
MVL	w1	1	2	2-1
BVR	w1	1	2,4	2-1
CJO	w1	1	4	2-1
IWB	w2	2	2	1
VVF	w2	2	2	2
NOL	w2	2	4	1
PHS	w2	2	4	1
CAA	w3	3	1,4	2
QBL (8W323)[*]	w3	3	2	2
HAR	w3	3	4	1
AVL	w3	3	4	1
BSM	w4	4	2	1
ATH	w5	5	2	2-1
WDV (8W149)	w6	w6	2,4	2-1
HHK	w6	w6	4	2
APD (8W148)	w6	w6	blank	2
DKB (8W324)	DB5	w9	4	1
VME	LDVII	blank	2	1

[*] between brackets: workshop numbers of the 8th International Histocompatibility Workshop.

lymphocytes from individuals which were SB4 negative, removing the
HLA-A, -B, -C and -DR antibodies. The reactivity of serum 34155 with
SB1 positive donors was eliminated by an additional absorption with
SB1 positive buffycoat lymphocytes. With the absorbed sera a panel
of 25 SB typed individuals was tested. Again an excellent correla-
tion with SB4 was observed (Table 4) (9).

Contradictory to expectation the SB4 specific antibodies reacted
almost exclusively with monocytes and not with B cells. This observation led to the question whether we were dealing with one of the
monocyte specific antigen systems previously described by Moraes
and Stastny (10) and Paul et al. (11). However, no similarity of
our sera with these systems was observed so far (data not shown).
As long as uncertainty exists on the identity of SB and the sero-
logically recognized gene products, we refer to the latter as
LB-F (9).

(3) The TCA system. The Tγ and Tµ cells, which probably have a

Table 4. Two by two comparison of SB4 with 5 different sera

SB4 serum no.	+ +	− +	+ −	− −	p *
37270	15	1	0	9	<0.0001
35572	15	1	0	9	<0.0001
34155	15	1	0	9	<0.0001
30147	15	8	0	2	0.15
1950	11	1	4	9	0.003

* Fisher's exact p value.

suppressor and helper function respectively, are cells which in the mouse have been shown to carry polymorphic determinants. We were interested to know whether we could identify such a polymorphism in man as well. Again the HLA-CAP approach was used in which sera from HLA-A1-B8-DR3 positive parous women were tested on lymphocytes from HLA-A1-B8-DR3 homozygous individuals. The T cells were separated in a Tγ and a Tμ enriched population using theophylline. This treatment renders the T cells much more sensitive for cytotoxicity. The most promising sera were selected and absorbed with Epstein-Barr virus transformed B cell-lines from the husband of the serum producer, to remove all anti-HLA-A, -B, -C and -DR antibodies. The absorbed sera were tested against a random panel. Like depicted in Figure 1, two independent diallelic systems could be identified. The TCA sera are mainly reactive with Tγ cells, the TCB sera with Tμ cells (12). Family studies further indicated that the TCA system might be encoded by a gene linked to HLA, located on the telomeric side of HLA-A. The lod-scores and recombination fraction of the total material of 9 families is given in Table 5. The fact that we could show that the TCA molecule is associated with β_2 microglobulin and has a molecular weight of 42 000 daltons (Giphart unpublished observations) implies that TCA might be equivalent to either Qa or TLA in the mouse. These antigens are biochemically similar to class I antigens but since they are only expressed on subpopulations of T cells, whereas class I antigens are expressed on all nucleated cells, they are rather referred to as class IV antigens (13). No genetic or biochemical data on the TCB system are available yet.

Linkage of T-cell alloantigens to HLA has been suggested by both Gazit et al. (14) for the activated T-cell differentiation markers designated by them as HT, and by Ferrara et al. (15). Okada et al. (16) encountered an anti T-cell serum reactive with T-suppressor cells (16). The relationships, if any, between these antigens and those described here remain to be determined.

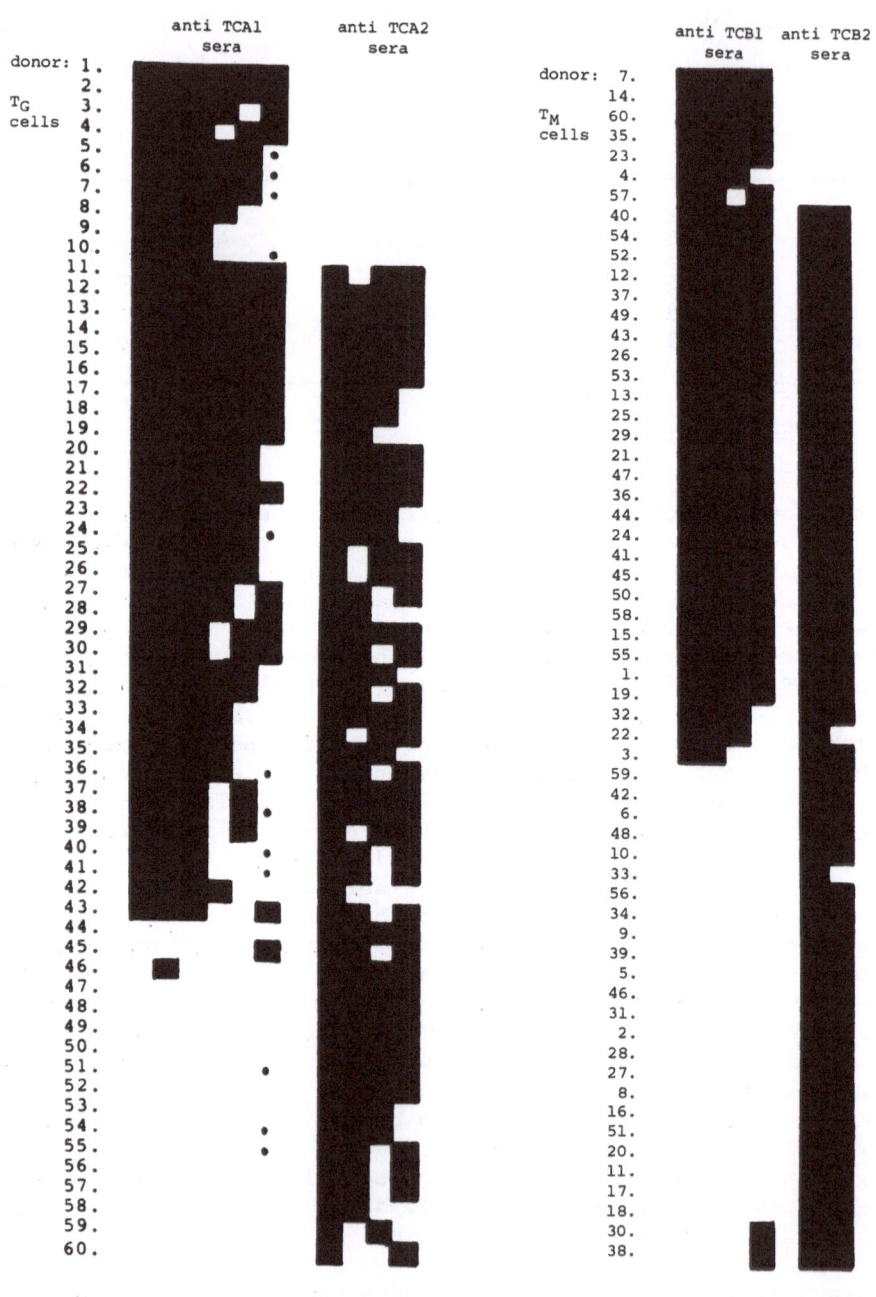

Fig. 1.   Reactions of 10 anti-TCA and 6 anti-TC8 sera with a panel
          of T-cell subsets obtained from unrelated donors.

Table 5. Lod (Z1) scores for nine informative families
          tested for T-cell system TCA and HLA haplotypes

recombination fraction						
0.05	0.10	0.15	0.20	0.25	0.30	0.40
−0.747	+0.675	+1.193	+1.324	+1.239	+1.018	+0.384

DISCUSSION AND SUMMARY

     For the recognition of "new" loci the HLA-CAP approach is impor-
tant and can be used for both humoral and cellular techniques. First,
with PLT cells raised in HLA-D/DR identical or compatible responder-
stimulator combinations, the SB/PL3 system was identified. Next,
the HLA-CAP approach combined with the use of the two colour fluorescence technique enabled us to identify sera which reacted with
different subpopulations of cells. Manipulation of antigenic sites
with theophylline and the use of ethidium bromide instead of eosine
as an indicator of cell death increased the sensitivity of the antibody detection. In this manner not only antisera reacting with
SB/PL3 determinants, but also antisera recognizing two different
systems of T cell polymorphisms could be identified: the TCA system
present on Tγ cells and most likely linked to HLA, and the TCB system, present on Tμ cells, but not yet genetically mapped.

     Our present view on the HLA supergene is given in Figure 2. The
class I antigens HLA-A, -B, -C and possibly TCA on the telomeric
side, the class II antigens HLA-D/DR, -MB/-DC1 LB-E (17,18,19) and

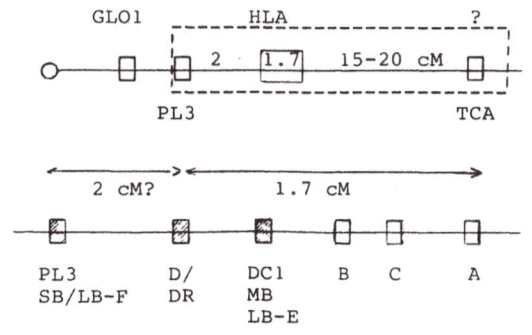

Fig. 2. The expending HLA supergene.

-SB/PL3 on the centromeric side. The red cell enzyme glyoxalase
(GLO1) is located between HLA and the centromere.

REFERENCES

1. Termijtelen, A., Bradley, B.A. and van Rood, J.J., Tissue
    Antigens 15:267 (1980).
2. Termijtelen, A. and van Rood, J.J., Tissue Antigens 17:57 (1981).
3. Shaw, S., Johnson, A.H. and Shearer, G.M., J. Exp. Med. 152:565
    (1980).
4. Mawas, C., Charmot, D., Sivy, M., Mercier, P., North, M.L. and
    Hauptmann, G., J. Immunogenet 5:383 (1978).
5. Shaw, S., Kavathas, P., Pollack, M.S., Charmot, D. and Mawas,
    C., Nature 293:745 (1981).
6. Nadler, L.M., Stashenko, P., Hardy, R., Pesando, J.M., Yunis,
    E.J. and Schlossman, S.F., Human Immunol. 1:77 (1981).
7. Shaw, S., DeMars, R., Schlossman, S.F., Smith, P.L., Lampson,
    L.A. and Nadler, L.M., Submitted for publication.
8. Van Rood, J.J., van Leeuwen, A. and Ploem, J.S., Nature 262:795
    (1976).
9. Van Leeuwen, A., Termijtelen, A. and Rood, J.J., Nature 298:565
    (1982).
10. Moraes, J.R. and Stastny, P., J. Clin. Invest. 60:449 (1977).
11. Paul, L.C., Claas, F.H.J., van Es, L.A., Kalff, M.W. and
    de Graeff, J., N. Engl. J. Med. 300:1258 (1979).
12. Van Leeuwen, A., Festenstein, H. and van Rood, J.J., Human
    Immunol. 4:109 (1982).
13. Snell, G.D., Science 213:172 (1981).
14. Gazit, E., Terhost, C. and Yunis, E.J., Nature 284:275 (1980).
15. Ferrara, G.B., Longo, A., Colombatti, M. and Moretta, L.,
    Human Immunol. 3:85 (1981).
16. Okada, J. and Stastny, P., Immunogenetics 16:59 (1982).
17. Duquesnoy, R.J., Marrari, M. and Annen, K., Transpl. Proc.
    11:1757 (1979).
18. Schreuder, G.M.Th., van Leeuwen, A., Termijtelen, A., Parlevliet,
    J., D'Amaro, J. and Rood, J.J., Human Immunol. 4:301 (1982).

MOLECULAR CLONING OF H-2 CLASS I GENES IN THE H-2[b] HAPLOTYPE

A.L. Mellor,[1] L. Golden,[1] E. Weiss,[1] H. Bullman,[1]
H. Bud,[1] J. Hurst,[1] R. Flavell,[1] R.F.L. James,[2]
E. Simpson,[3] A.R.M. Townsend,[4] P.M. Taylor,[4]
J. Ferluga,[5] L. Leben,[5] M. Santamaria,[5] G. Atfield,[5]
and H. Festenstein[5]

Laboratory of Gene Structure and Expression, National
Institute for Medical Research. The Ridgeway, Mill Hill,
London NW7 1AA, UK[1]; ICRF Tumour Immunology Unit,
University College, Gower Street, London WC1E 6 BT, UK[2];
Clinical Research Centre, Watford Road, Harrow, Middlesex
HA1 3UJ, UK[3]; Division of Immunology, National Institute
for Medical Research, The Ridgeway, Mill Hill, London
NW7 1AA, UK[4]; Dept. of Immunology, the London Hospital
Medical School, University of London, Turner Street,
London E1 2AD, UK[5].

We have cloned H-2 class I genes of the C57BL/10 (B10, H-2[b]
haplotype) mouse using cosmid cloning techniques developed in our

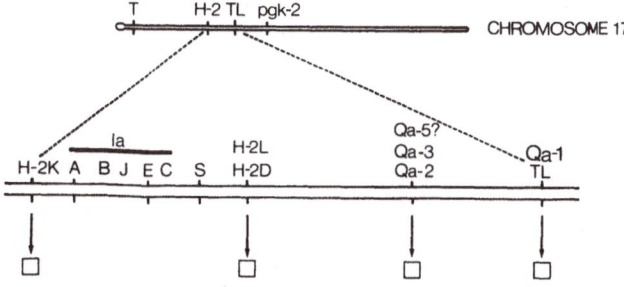

Fig. 1. Genetic Map of H-2 and associated loci on chromosome 17.
The four loci known to control the expression of H-2
class I antigens are indicated (□).

69

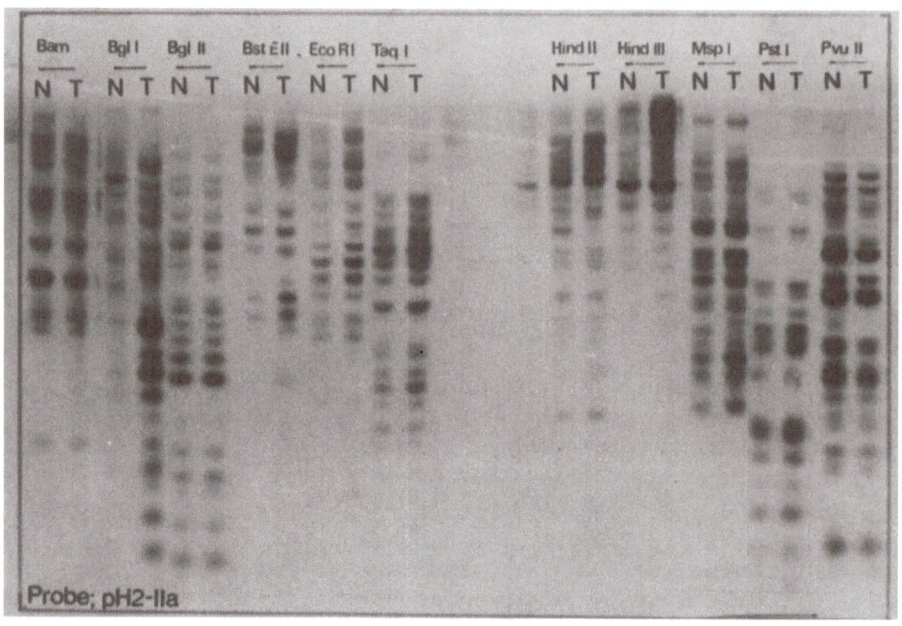

Fig. 2. Autoradiograph showing hybridisation patterns of mouse
class I DNA cDNA probe (pH2-IIa, obtained from Dr. M.
Steinmetz) on Mouse spleen DNA's digested with various
restriction enzymes. Names of restriction enzymes are given
above each pair of tracks. N=AKR spleen DNA. T=AKR spontaneous tumor DNA.

laboratory (1). Cosmids, which contain 40-45 kilobasepairs (kbp) of
mouse DNA per clone, were chosen since there are about 20-30 class
I genes (see below) in the mouse genome and most of these genes map
between the H-2K and TL loci on chromosome 17 (Figure 1); a region
of some 1000 kbp. of DNA. Estimates of the number of class I genes
in the mouse genome are based on Southern blot analysis (2) in
which restriction enzyme digested mouse genomic DNA is hybridised
to a class I H-2 cDNA probe (Figure 2). In all digests shown, and
in all three H-2 haplotypes tested, the cDNA probe hybridises to
multiple bands in the digests indicating that the H-2 class I are
multiple copy and highly homologous. Using either H-2 cDNA or H-LA
genomic probes we have isolated 90 cosmids containing class I genes
from a mouse genomic library constructed using B10 spleen DNA. These
cosmids have been organised into 5 distinct clusters of overlapping
mouse DNA on the basis of restriction enzyme mapping and Southern
blot hybridisation analysis (Table 1). The DNA regions cloned in
each cosmid cluster have been mapped to one of the four genetic loci
known, from immunological analysis, to control the expression of
class I cell surface antigens in the B10 mouse (see Figure 1). To
assign specific DNA regions to specific genetic loci, we exploited

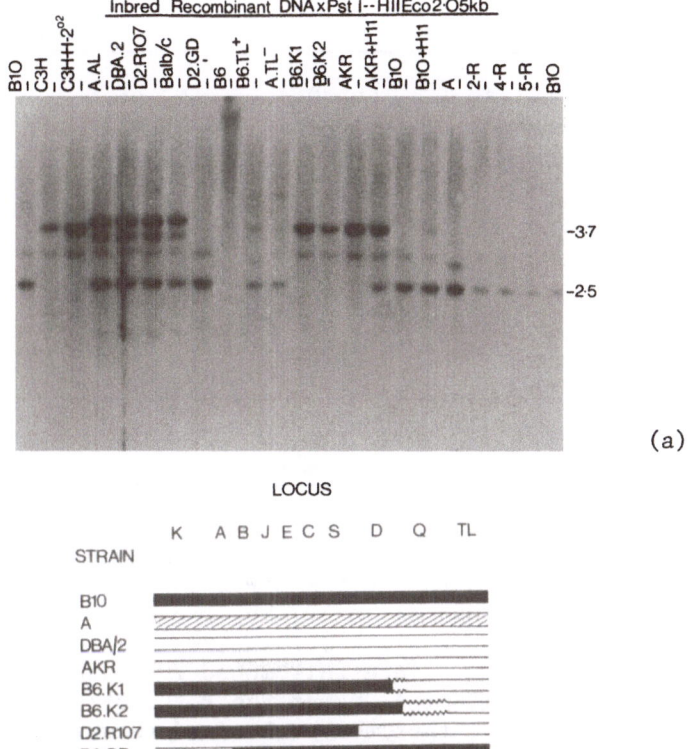

(a)

(b)

Fig. 3a. Autoradiograph showing hybridization pattern obtained
          when a 2.05kb EcoRI fragment from cosmid H11 is used as
          a hybridization probe on Pst I digested spleen DNA
          extracted from various inbred mice. Sizes of bands in
          B10 (2.5 kilobases), AKR and B6.K2 (3.7 kilobases) are
          shown on the right.

Fig. 3b. Schematic diagrams showing origin of DNA in various H-2
          recombinant inbred strains and the positions of recombina-
          tions in the DNA with respect to the genetic map of the
          H-2 region.

the extensive restriction enzyme polymorphisms which are detected
between different H-2 inbred strains of mice using a Southen blotting
procedure. Unique mouse DNA fragments (which therefore do not contain
class I gene sequences, or mouse repetitive DNA elements) were isolated from each cosmid cluster and used as hybridisation probes on
total digested DNA from H-2^b (B10 or B6), H-2^d (Balb/c), H-2^k (AKR)
and H-2 recombinant inbred mouse strains. Strain specific restriction
enzyme polymorphisms can thus be used to map hybridising bands to
specific genetic loci defined by recombinant inbred mouse strains.

Table 1. The organisation of cosmids

Cosmid Cluster	N° of Class I Genes	Kbp DNA Cloned	N° of Cosmids	Genetic Locus
1	2	90	7	H-2K
2	1	40	2	H-2D
3	5	120	15	Qa2,3
4	2	60	2	Qa2,3 or TL
5	5	120	39	TL
Total	15	430	65	

For example, a unique 2.05 kbp DNA probe isolated from cosmid H11
in cluster 5 hybridises to a 2.5 kbp Pst I fragment in digests of
B10, A and Balb/c DNA whereas a 3.7 kbp fragment is detected in the
AKR Pst-I digest (Figure 3a). A 3.7 kbp fragment is also detected
in digests of B6.K1 DNA. Since this mouse recombinant has AKR DNA
at the TL locus and B10 or A DNA at the H-2K, H-2D and Qa2.3 loci
(Figure 3b) we conclude that the probe (and therefore the mouse H-2
class I genes cloned in cosmid cluster 5) maps to the TL locus in
the B10 mouse.

    Most of the class I genes cloned in the cosmid clusters map to
either the Qa2,3 or to the T1 loci (Table 1). This result is surprising given the extreme polymorphism of the antigens expressed at the
H-2K and H-2D loci. Nevertheless, it is possible that the class I
genes mapping to the Qa-2,3 and TL loci are involved in the generation of H-2 polymorphism, by means of unequal gene pairing and gene
conversion (3). We are currently investigating the mechanism of H-2

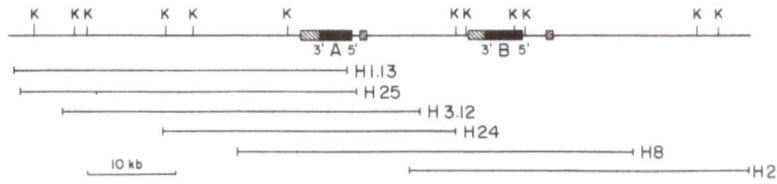

Fig. 4.   Gene organization in cluster 1 which maps to the H-2K
          locus. Two closely linked gene regions, A and B, are
          arranged head to tail (5'→ 3'). K = KpnI restriction
          sites. Extent of cosmids defining this region is shown
          under the map.

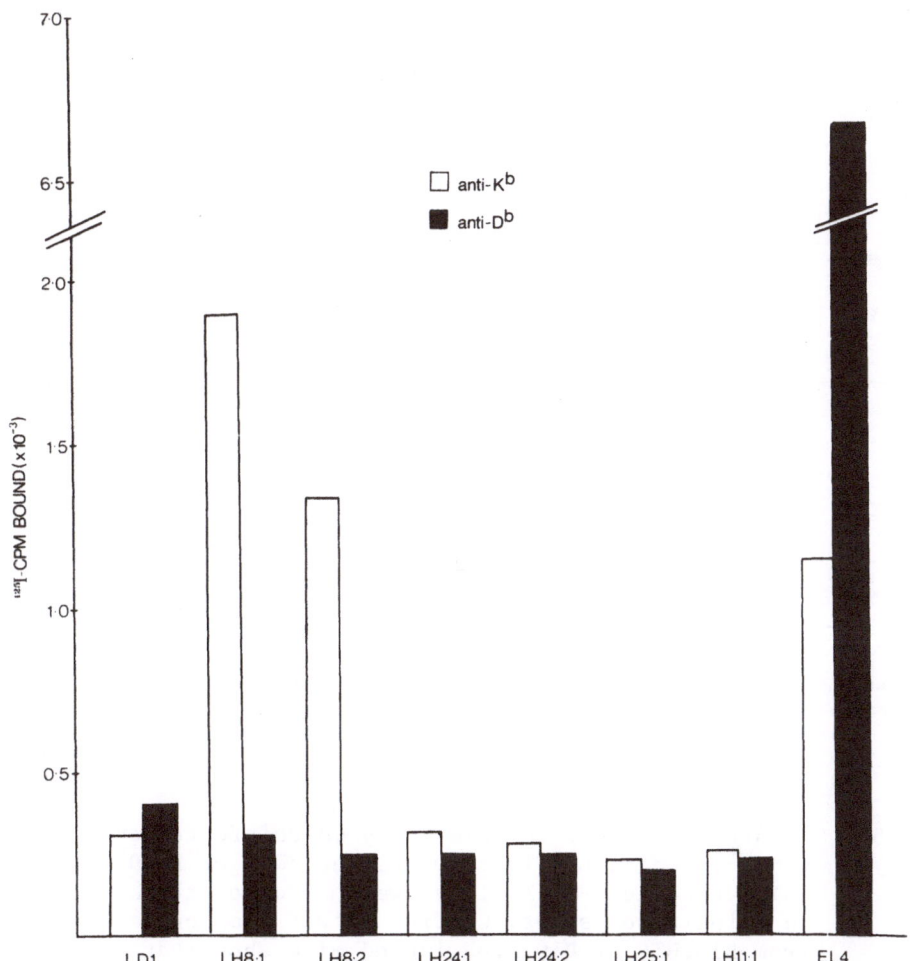

Fig. 5a. Radioimmunoassay to detect H–2K^b (□) or H–2D^b (■)
antigens on the surface of cosmid transformed cell lines.
Monoclonal antibodies against H–2K^b or H–2D^b were bound
to each cell line ^{125}I sheep anti-mouse Ig was bound
subsequently. LD1 – control untransformed L–cell line;
LH8.2, LH8.1 – cell lines transformed with cosmid H8;
LH24.1, LH24.2 – cell lines transformed with cosmid H24;
LH25.1, LH11.1 – cell lines transformed with cosmids H25,
and H11 respectively. EL4 – control H–2^b haplotype
lymphoma cell line.

polymorphism by cloning the altered class I antigens expressed at
the H–2K locus in the bm series of mouse mutants isolated by
Nathenson and co-workers (4).

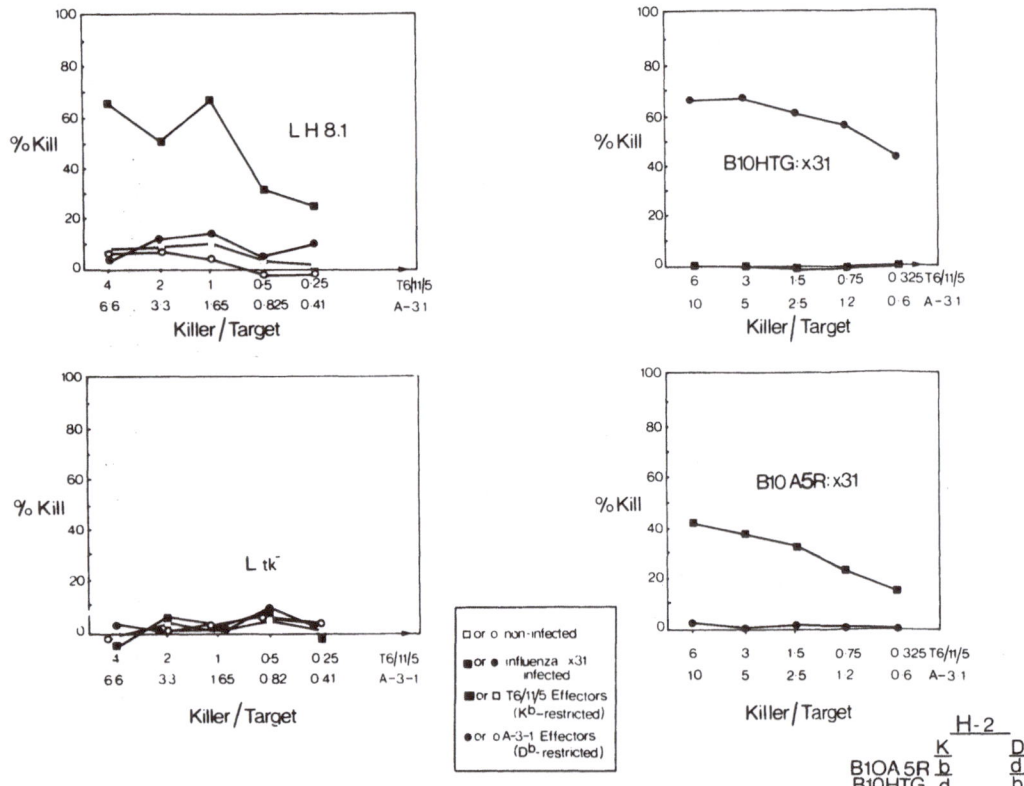

Fig. 5b. ^{51}Chromium (^{51}Cr) release assay on uninfected or influenza
virus infected LH8.1 or LD1 target cell or H-2D^b restrict-
ed) cytotoxic T-cell clones were used as attacker cells
in triplicate assays. Control target lymphocytes derived
from B10.HTG or B10.A.5R inbred mice show that the two
attacker T-cell clones have absolute requirements for
either H-2K^b or H-2D^b as restriction elements.

As well as determining the structure and organisation of the
cloned H-2 class I genes we have used cosmids to transform L-cells
(H-2^k haplotype) and tested the resulting transformants (using a
variety of immunological methods) for the presence of new H-2^b
haplotype specific cell surface antigens. Thus, by identifying a
particular class I, H-2^b antigen on the surface of transformed
L-cells we at once confirm the genetic mapping data presented above
and also generate cell lines which have a single H-2^b class I molecule on the cell surface. These lines will be useful in studying
class I gene expression and in defining the functions of class I
antigens in immune reactions. For example, cosmids from cluster 1
(Figure 4) define 2 class I gene regions separated by only 15 kbp.

When these cosmids are used to transform L-cells H-2K^b cell surface antigen appears on the surface of cells transformed with H8, and not with H24, H25 as determined by (i) monoclonal antibody binding (Figure 5a) (ii) antibody dependent, complement mediated lysis (iii) allogeneic T-cell lysis and (iv) influenza specific, H-2^b restricted T-cell lysis (Figure 5b). This suggests that gene B (Figure 4) encodes the H-2K^b antigen. We have confirmed this finding by using a subcloned DNA fragment, taken from cosmid H8, which contains only gene B. This subclone also causes H-2K^b expression in transformed L-cells as assayed by the above immunological tests. The function of gene A, if it is capable of expressing a class I like antigen, is unknown. We have also determined, using the same procedures, that H-2D^b is expressed on cells transformed with cosmids from cluster 2.

REFERENCES

1. Grosveld, F.G., Dahl, H.H.M., DeBoer, E. and Flavell, R.A., Gene 13:227 (1981).
2. Southern, E.M., J. Mol. Biol. 98:503 (1975).
3. Flavell, R.A., Bud, H., Bullman, H., Busslinger, M., DeBoer, E., deKleine, A., Golden, L., Groffen, J., Grosveld, F.G., Mellor, A.L., Moschonas, N., and Weiss, E., "Proceedings of 6th International Congress of Human Genetics", Israel (1981).
4. Nairn, R., Yamaga, K. and Nathenson, S.G., A Rev. Genet. 14:241-277 (1980).

WHY STUDY COMPLEMENT GENETICS?

Peter Lachmann

Medical Research Council, Mechanisms in Tumour
Immunity Unit, Cambridge, England

When Mallory was asked why he wished to climb Mount Everest he
answered "because it's there". Similarly complement genetics should
be studied because there is so much genetic variation there to study.
Table 1 shows how common genetic polymorphisms are among human complement components. The term "polymorphism" was coined by E.B.
Ford (1) to denote an allelic system where the second most common
allele occurs at a frequency too high to be maintained by mutation
alone (generally taken as a frequency above 1%). It is generally
held that polymorphisms are maintained in the population by selection, the heterozygote having some selective advantage to compensate
for any disadvantage of the less favourable allele. The classic example is the case of haemoglobin S where the heterozygote enjoys
some protection against death from malaria in the early months of
life, which compensates for the considerable disadvantage of homozygous sickle cell disease. It is with this example in mind that
the existence of the complement polymorphisms (and particularly of
high frequency polymorphisms where the frequency of the second
allele exceeds 10% -which occurs for C3, C6, Factor B and C4-) has
led to a long and hard search for functional differences between
the different alleles and for association of individual alleles with
diseases in man.

It must however be admitted that the general truth of the selectionist explanation for polymorphisms is not certainly established. It is, for example, quite possible that in some cases a
polymorphic locus is closely linked to a second polymorphic locus
where the polymorphism is maintained by selection. In this case the
polymorphism at the first locus will necessarily be maintained even
if there is no functional difference between its alleles.

Table 1.   Genetic Variation in Complement Proteins

	Polymorphism with second allele frequency (F)		Deficiency ([†])=relatively frequent
	F>10%	10%>F>1%	
C1q			X
C1r			X
C1s			(X)
C4	XX		X
C2		X	X[†](Caucasian)
C3	X		X
C5		(X) (Melanesians)	X
C6	X		X
C7		X	X
C8 α-γ		X	X
C8 β		X	X
C9			X[†](Japanese)
FB	X		
FD		X (Gambians)	
FP			X (X-linked)
1			X
H			X

It is furthermore conceivable that the selectionist explanation may sometimes be genuinely wrong and that variants which are quite neutral in their effects may persist in populations for reasons that have not so far been explained.

This may be the case with the polymorphisms of two closely linked complement components C6 and C7. In man C6 shows the most widespread high frequency polymorphism of all the complement components (Table 2). The second most frequent C6 allele occurs at a frequency of 35% in all the major human races. In spite of this striking polymorphism there is no obvious haemolytic difference between the two alleles and C6 is not known to have any functions other than its involvement in the haemolytic process. The closely linked locus for C7, which is the next acting component in the complement sequence, shows no common polymorphism in man although rare variants have been described that allow the locus to be mapped. C6 and C7 polymorphisms have now also been studied in a number of other mammalian species and in some birds. Polymorphisms of both components have been found and the results obtained in mammals by Eldridge and Hobart (2) are shown in Table 3. They show that either or both or neither of C6 and C7 may show polymorphisms in different mammalian species. Many of the species studied were different vari-

Table 2. Unassigned Complement Loci (3-6)

Component	HLA Linkage Excluded by	Gene Frequency (Structural Variants)	Commonest	Second	Others
C1R	Deficiency	No Data			
C3	Allotypes Deficiency	Caucasoids Mongoloids Negroids	0.77 0.99 0.93	0.22 <0.01 0.06	Rare
C5	Deficiency	Caucasoids and Negroids	Very Low or Absent (0/2262)		
C6	Allotypes Deficiency	All Races	0.6	0.35	0.05
C7	Allotypes Deficiency	Caucasoids	0.99	<0.01	<0.01
C8	Allotypes Deficiency	Negroids	0.99	6 Rare	
Factor D	No Data	Negroids	0.98	0.02	

Table 3.   Numbers of Species (Mammals) (7)

| | | C6 Polymorphism | | |
		+	−	Assay Failed
C7 Polymorphism	+	4	5	0
	−	8	8	1
	Assay Failed	4	3	

eties of large cat and are otherwise quite closely related. It is
difficult to put forward a selective explanation for these polymorphisms in the face of their random distribution in closely related
species and one may suspect that they are indeed neutral in their
effect.

The situation is quite different with C3. Here the second most
common allele, C3f shows a markedly different distribution in different racial groups and is in fact appreciably common only among
Caucasians where it is found with a frequency of 22% (Table 2). C3f
also shows functional differences from the common allele C3s, having
a higher capacity to form rosettes with macrophages (8) and probably
a lower specific haemolytic activity. It has furthermore been reported by McLean (9,10) that there is an increased frequency of the
C3f allele in patients with mesangiocapillary glomerulo-nephritis,
with partial lipodystrophy and with juvenile systemic lupus erythe-
matosis. It is of interest that these are the very same diseases
that are associated with the occurence of nephritic factor, the
autoantibody which reacts with C3b, B and it may be tempting to
postulate that C3f is more "antigenic" for the formation of this
autoantibody than other alleles of C3. It is likely that there is
some compensating selective advantage for having C3f, perhaps associated with its higher rosetting ability and it seems reasonable
to conclude that C3 polymorphism is maintained by a balanced selective process.

With regard to the HLA-linked complement locus, the situation
is clearly highly complex since the complement polymorphisms here
are in close linkage with other highly polymorphic loci and this
will be discussed later in the symposium by Dr Hauptmann.

Table 4. Complement Loci

Components	Linkage Data
C4, C2, Factor B	Very close to B locus of HLA
C6, C7	Unassigned
C3	Loose linkage to Lewis Blood groups (N.B. In mice loose linkage to H-2)
C1 C5 C8 Factor D C1̄ inhibitor C3b inactivator	Unassigned and show no linkage to any of the three loci above (Insufficient data to exclude linkage within this group of components)

WHAT USE CAN BE MADE OF COMPLEMENT POLYMORPHISMS?

Gene Mapping by Pedigree Analysis

The classical techniques of gene mapping by family analysis have demonstrated three major complement loci and a number of minor ones. These are listed in table 4. The three loci where there is ample mapping data are the HLA-linked locus for C2, C4 and Factor B; the as yet unassigned locus for C6 and C7; and the locus for C3 now known to be on chromosome 19. These three loci are clearly known not to be linked to each other and none of them shows linkage to any of the other loci shown. Whether any of these less completely known loci show any linkage to each other is not certainly known. This technique can sometimes be applied not only to family pedigrees, but to those

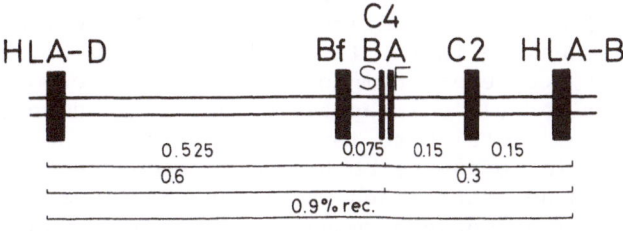

Fig. 1. The HLA-linked Complement loci

Table 5.   Allotype Conversion after liver transplantation
           in Man (11)

Shown to occur for:		Shown not to occur for:
C3	Gc-globulin	IgG
C6	Haptoglobulin	
C8	Orosomucoid	
Factor B	Transferrin	
	αl-antitrypsin	

entire populations where the number of founder chromosomes was small.
Olaisen (12) has recently studied the complement allotypes in the
HLA region in a Scandinavian population which has been stable for
many centuries and by counting the crossovers from the putative
founder chromosomes has been able to suggest an order for the HLA-
linked complement components which is shown in Figure 1. The order
is somewhat surprising since C4 is found to lie between Factor B
(Bf) and C2, two components that are certainly gene duplicates. It
will be interesting to see in due course if DNA analysis gives the
same answer.

Paternity Testing

     Some complement allotypes e.g. C6 and C3 occur at a sufficient-
ly high frequency to be useful for paternity testing. Although this
is of limited scientific interest it provides a source of funds for
the allotyping laboratories.

Allotype Conversion Studies

     The existence of high frequency polymorphisms leads to the sit-
uation where organ grafts -and particularly liver grafts- are carried out in situations where the donor and recipient show different
alleles. This allows one to determine whether the serum component
involved is synthesised in the liver. Such studies have been done
for a variety of complement components and other serum proteins
largely by Alper and his colleagues (6) and have shown (see Table 5)
that all the serum proteins so far tested with the sole exception
of IgG, and this includes the complement components C3, C6, Factor B
and C8, appear to be synthesised wholly by the liver. This is shown
by the total and apparently permanent conversion to donor allotype
after liver transplantation. This can further be used as evidence
that it is the hepatocytes and not the Kupffer cells that synthesize

Table 6. Families of Complement Components

	Complement			
Family defined principally by:	Classical Pathway	Alternative Pathway	Membrane Attack Complex	Others
Hydrazine sensitivity				
Proteolytic activation	C4	C3	C5	Alpha 2 – macroglobulin
– Anaphylotoxins				
Heat lability				
Zymogens of complex and unusual serine esterases	C2 ———— FB		(C6) – (C7)	
Inhibitability by C1-inhibitor	C1r, C1s	(FD)		F XIIa F XIa Kallikrein Plasmin

Components joined by lines show genetic linkage in man

Factors XIIa and XI of the coagulation system. If the capacity to
be inhibited by C1-inhibitor does indeed demonstrate a common evolutionary origin —and this will require structural evidence in due
course— then one might conclude, as it is indeed attractive to speculate for other reasons, that the initiation protease of the classical
complement pathway shares a common evolutionary origin with the contact activatable pathways. Whether Factor D of the alternative pathway, which is not inhibited by C1-inhibitor is in fact a further
'deviant' member of the same family, is uncertain, but it serves one
of the functions in the alternative pathway that C1 serves in the
classical pathway. Further analysis of these family relations would
be helped by genetic information on all the components. Whereas the
phenotypic genetic studies by pedigree analysis that I have so far
discussed can be expected to continue to give valuable information,
there is little doubt that in future an increasingly powerful tool
for these as for other genetic studies will be the use of 'genomic
genetics', studying the genes directly by the techniques of recombinant DNA technology. For one complement component, C3, this work
is already well established in the laboratory of Dr. George Fey who
will bring us up to date on this exciting and new field.

Beside the structural polymorphisms of complement component
there is a further type genetic variation now found for nearly all
complement components and these are the isolated deficiencies. These
isolated deficiencies are of particular value in allowing the functions of complex systems like complement to be studied in vivo as
opposed to simply in the test tube, by observing the consequences
of the absence of particular components. A propos of human studies
it is worth making the point that the associations found may be due
not to the consequences of the complement deficiency itself, but
either to ascertainment artefact or to closely linked genes which
carry the susceptibilities to the diseases which are observed. It
is now possible to be fairly certain that the associations particularly of immune complex disease with complement deficiency are not
due to ascertainment artefacts. There are enough studies of complement deficiencies in normal populations to be able to calculate a
crude estimate of average relative risk for such associations and
for the association of S.L.E. with C2 deficiency it is in the region
of 50. However the possibility that the disease associations are
due to linked genes cannot be generally discarded and in the HLA
region in particular the possibility is always there. However the
observation that certain diseases such as mesangiocapillary glomeru-
lonephritis are associated with a particular allele of C3 and with
deficiency of C6 (which are unlinked loci); and that S.L.E. is associated not only with deficiencies of C2 and C4, but also with
that of C1 and with hereditary angio-oedema (where deficiencies of
C2 and C4 are secondary to the deficiency of C1-inhibitor because
of unrestrained catabolism) are strong evidence that the association
is physiological.

these proteins, since the Kupffer cells are believed to be replaced
from bone marrow derived cells and should gradually revert to host
type.

Gene Duplication and Complement Evolution

I have argued more fully elsewhere that the complement system
has developed from simpler precursors by progressive gene duplication. The duplications responsible for the generation of the complement system as we know it must all have happened a long way back in
phylogeny. However, it is clear that complement component loci still
duplicate and the information on this topic is derived from largely
allotype studies. It is widely known that the C4 locus in man is
duplicated and Dr. Hauptmann will enlarge on this matter. It is
perhaps less widely known that C7 locus, which in man we have every
reason to think is a single locus, is duplicated both in the
dog (2), and in Przewalski's horse (3). One can be fairly sure that
the duplications in the dog and Przewalski's horse are separate
events. This must show that duplication of loci for complement components is not particularly rare, but even in reasonable recent
evolutionary time it has occurred, on more than one occasion, even
for a single component.

Families of Complement Components

The realisation that complement components occur in families
which arose by this process of gene duplication makes the complexities of complement easier to understand. There are now three reasonably well established families which are listed in Table 6. The most
important and most fascinating of these families is that which comprises C3, C4 and C5, to which alpha 2 macroglobulin must now be
added. It has been found in recent years that these proteins (or at
least three of them) have the capacity to attach covalently to acceptor structures by a transacylation reaction involving the cleavage of an internal thioester bond. This family is discussed in
detail by Dr. Harrison. The family comprising Factor B and C2 is
also well established. These are the zymogens of the complex serine
esterases that make up the C3-clearing enzymes of the alternative
and classical pathways of the complement system. C6, which has recently been shown also to have one of the features of a serine esterase in being inhibitable by DFP (14) and therefore also its
presumed gene duplicate C7 may represent further members of the same
family. This would make sense since in its reaction pattern C6
stands in the same relation to C5 as Factor B does to C3 or C2 does
to C4. The third family can perhaps best be defined by the capacity
of the enzymes which it comprises to be inhibited by the $\overline{C1}$-
inhibitor. This definition would include not only the two sub-
components of C1, C1r and C1s, but also plasmin and kallikrein and

because of unrestrained catabolism) are strong evidence that the
association is physiological.

For all the reasons given above therefore there seems good
reason to take an interest in the genetics of the complement system
in the data which will be given in the succeeding talks.

REFERENCES

1. Ford, E.B., in: "Genetics for Medical Students", Methuen,
    London (1942).
2. Eldridge, P.R., Hobart, M.J. and Lachmann, P.J., in:
    "Biochemical Genetics" (1982)(in press).
3. Vas Guedes, M.A., Hobart, M.J. and Lachmann, P.J.,
    J. Immunogenet. 5:279-282 (1978).
4. Alper, C.A., Hobart, M.J. and Lachmann, P.J., in: "Isoelectric
    Focusing", Arbuthnott, J.P. and Beeley, J.A. (eds.), pp. 306-312,
    Butterworths, London (1975).
5. Mittal, K.K., Wolski, K.P., Lim, D., Gewurz, A., Gewurz, H. and
    Schmidt, F.R., Tissue Antigens 7:97-104 (1976).
6. Rittner, C., Opferkuch, W., Weleek, B., Grosse-Wilde, H. and
    Wernet, P., Human Genet. 34:137-142 (1976).
7. Eldridge, P.R. and Hobart, M.J., cited in Lachmann, P.J. and
    Hobart, M.J., in: "The genetics of the complement system",
    Ciba Found. Symp. 66:231 (1979).
8. Arvilommi, H., Nature (Lond.) 251:740-741 (1974).
9. Mclean, R.H. and Hoefnagel, D., Hum. Hered. 30:149 (1980).
10. McLean, R.H., Abeles, M., Weinstein, A., Kennedy, T.L. and
    Rothfield, N., Ann. Rheum. Assoc. Ann. Sci. Meet. Atlanta (1980).
11. Alper, C.A., Raum, D., Awdeh, Z.L., Petersen, B.H., Taylor, P.D.
    and Starzl, T.E., Clin. Immunol. Immunopathol. 16:84-89 (1980).
12. Olaisen, B., Teisberg, P. and Gedde-Dahl, T., Jr., Personal
    Communication (1982).
13. Whitehouse, D., Personal Communication (1982).
14. Kolb, W.P., Kolb, L.M. and Savary, J.R., Biochem 21:294-301
    (1982).

THE FAMILY OF PROTEINS HAVING INTERNAL THIOLESTER BONDS

R.A. Harrison

Medical Research Council Centre
Cambridge, England

Historic Perspective and Development of the Concept of an Internal Thiolester Bond

It is over fifty years since the complement component C4 was first described as being ammonia and hydrazine sensitive (1). Ecker, Pillemer and Seifter (2) later confirmed this sensitivity of C4 to nitrogen nucleophiles, and in 1953 both a plasmatic inhibitor of serum and "Factor A" of the properdin pathway were shown to be inactivated by hydrazine (3,4). However, it was not until 1968 that the plasmatic inhibitor was identified as α_2-macroglobulin and 1972 that the hydrazine-sensitive factor of the properdin or alternative pathway of complement was shown to be C3 (5,6).

While treatment of C4 with hydrazine was shown to inhibit binding to membranes or immune complexes, the statement that this interaction was "probably covalent" (7) was not experimentally justified until much later. However, these plasma proteins are now known to be capable, on activation, of forming covalent bonds to seemingly unrelated molecules. The first convincing demonstration of this was shown in the interaction of α_2-macroglobulin and plasmin (8,9). The complex formed resisted disruption in sodium dodecyl sulphate, but did not involve the active site serine hydroxyl of the protease and was therefore different from that between other potease inhibitors and proteases (e.g. α_1-protease inhibitor and trypsin (10). The first demonstration of a covalent bond involving a complement component was that of C3b to membranes (11). This observation was later extended to the interaction of C4b with membranes (12) and the interaction of both C4b and C3b with immunoglobulin (13,14).

Parallel with this work were investigations into the chemical

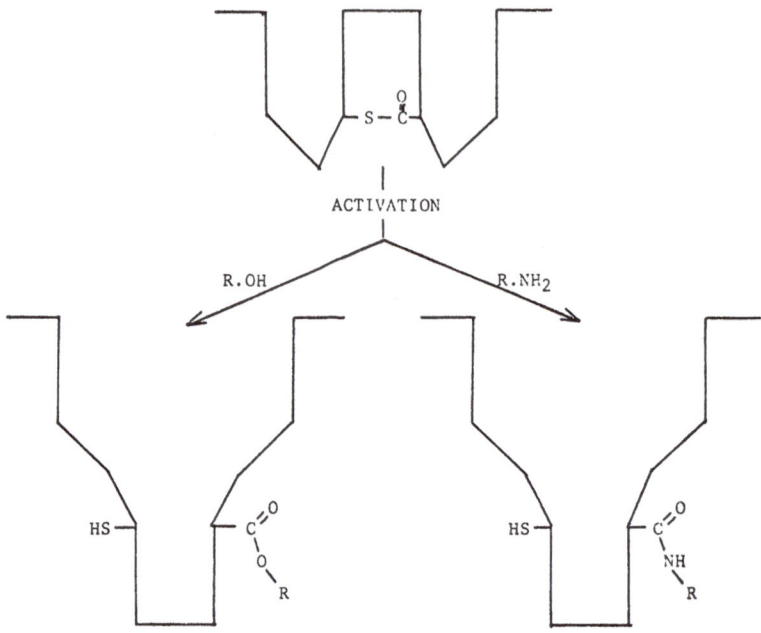

Fig. 1.   Thiolester-containing proteins possess a reactive acyl group
          that confers the potential for ester and/or amide bond form-
          ation with receptive molecules. The reactive acyl group is
          susceptible to attack by small nitrogen nucleophiles with
          concomitant release of a single thiol group.

basis of the nucleophile sensitivity of these proteins. Investigation
of the reaction conditions of hydroxylamine with C4 led Seifter,
Katchalski and Harkness (15) to suggest that inactivation was caused
by nucleophilic attack at an ester. More recently, Law, Lichtenberg
and Levine (16), studying the interaction of C3b with membranes, suggested that an activated acyl or amide group might exist in the native
protein (C3) and, on activation, an oxyester bond be formed between
C3b and a surface hydroxyl group by a transacylation reaction. At the
same time, a specific methylamine-reactive glutamyl residue was re-
cognised in α_2-macroglobulin (17). Both these groups suggested that
one way in which an acyl group could be activated was, in accord with
earlier deductions of Seifter and coworkers, as an internal ester.
However, the key observation was that of Janatova and coworkers, who
showed that nucleophile inactivation, chaotroph inactivation and
proteolytic activation of C3 all led to the stoichiometric release
of a single thiol (18). This enabled these workers and others to
postulate that the acyl group was activated as an internal thiolester,
and that covalent bonds between thiolester-containing proteins and
acceptor molecules were formed when this acyl group was transferred
to an acceptor hydroxyl group. The interaction of C3b and C4b with

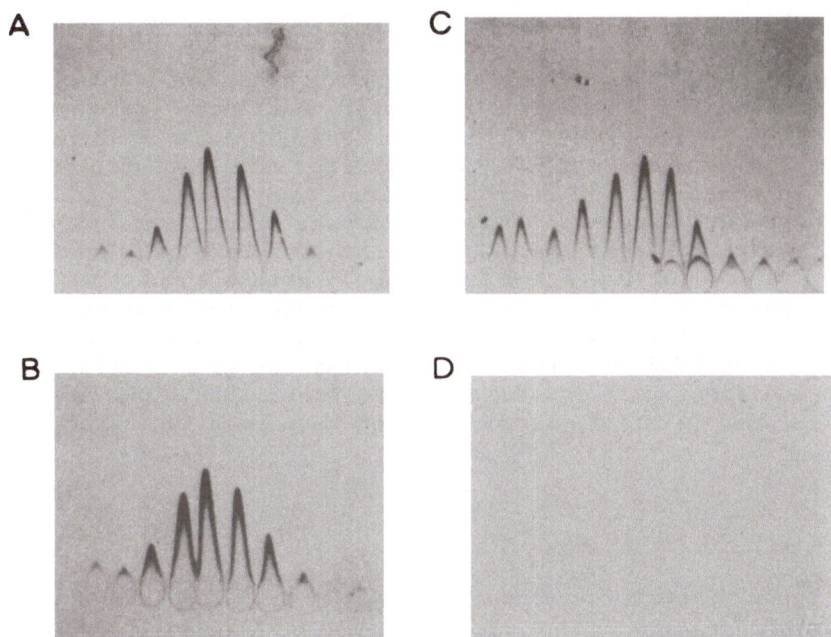

Fig. 2.   Identification of α_2-Macroglobulin as a Thiolester-Containing
          Protein.
          All four panels show single dimension crossed immunoelectro-
          phoresis of DEAE-Sephacel column fractions into anti α_2-
          macroglobulin. Panels A and C show the Coomassie-stained
          plate and B and D the corresponding autoradiographs.
          A, B - Plasma treated with 14C-iodoacetamide in the presence
          of methylamine. C, D - Plasma treated with 14C-iodoacetamide
          in the absence of methylamine.

immunoglobulin is now known to involve hydroxylamine-resistant as
well as hydroxylamine-sensitive or oxyester bonds. These are thought
to be amide bonds and to be formed by transfer of the activated acyl
group to an acceptor amino group (13,14). Less is known about the
interaction between α_2-macroglobulin and proteases. However, a correlation between the lysine content of the protease and the efficiency of covalent bond formation suggests that here also amide bonds
might be formed (19,20).

These concepts are shown schematically in Figure 1. With all
three proteins, treatment with nitrogen nucleophiles abolishes the
potential for covalent bond formation.

Identification of Thiolester-Containing Plasma Proteins

We have used the nucleophile-dependent release of a thiol as a
method for scanning plasma for thiolester-containing proteins. The
protocol used is summarised as follows: Freshly drawn EDTA-plasma
was treated with iodoacetamide to block free thiol groups, dialysed
to remove unreacted iodoacetamide, and then divided into two portions. These were incubated with ^{14}C-iodoacetamide, one in the presence of methylamine and the other in the absence of the nucleophile.
Following removal of unreacted radiolabel, both were chromatographed
on DEAE-Sephacel and column fractions monitored for nucleophile-
specific uptake of iodoacetamide. Using this procedure α_2-macroglo-
bulin was identified as a thiolester-containing protein (Figure 2).
(21). In addition, at least two proteins other than those currently
known (i.e. C3, C4 and α_2-macroglobulin) have been indicated but not
yet identified.

The Structure of the Thiolester Site

Nucleophile-specific release of a thiol from thiolester-containing proteins has also been used in the specific isolation of peptides
containing the reactive acyl and thiol groups. After activation the
protein under investigation was immobilised on activated thiol-
Sepharose, digested with a protease, the released peptides washed
from the matrix, and the thiol-containing peptide finally released
by cysteine or dithiothreitol. This approach has several attractive
features, notably selection of protease and digestion conditions (no
cleavage between the reactive acyl group and the liberated thiol) on
a small aliquot of immobilised protein and single step fractionation
from both released peptides and protease. In addition, the use of a
radio-labelled nucleophile (^{14}C-methylamine) during activation per-
mits ascertainment of the position of the reactive acyl group, ascertainment of the stoichiometry of thiol release (using ^{3}H-iodoacetic
acid) and confirmation of the position of the reactive acyl group
relative to the Sepharose-bound thiol. The amino acid sequences
around the thiolester sites in both C3 (21) and C4 (22) have been
determined using this approach. In Figure 3 these sequences are compared with that of α_2-macroglobulin. It is immediately apparent that
there is considerable sequence homology, particularly carboxy-terminal
to the thiolester site. (It is possible that the conserved region at
the carboxy-terminal end of the sequences shown and beginning at
tyr-40, while of interest in indicating an ancestral relationship
between these proteins, may not relate to structural requirements
for a thiolester but rather to a potential for carbohydrate attach-
ment.) The penta-peptide sequence -gly-cys-gly-glu-glu- is totally
conserved and contains both the reactive acyl group, glu-26, and the
thiol released on activation, cys-23. Model building studies (26)
have shown that these two groups can indeed bridge to form a thiolester, strengthening the hypothesis that such a bond exists in the

```
           5        10        15        20        25        30        35        40        45        50
C3:  A Q M T E D A V D A E R L K H L I V T P S G C G E E N M I G M T P T V I A V S Y L B E T E Q W E K
C4:    G S E G A L S P G G V A S L L R L P R G C G E E T M I Y L A P T L A A S R Y L D K T E Q X X X L
α₂M:  V L G D I L G S A M Q N T Q N L L Q M P Y G C G E E N M V L F A P N I Y V L D Y L N E T Q Q L T P E
```

C3 - Thomas et al, 1982.
C4 - Campbell et al, 1981; Harrison et al, 1981.
α₂M - Swenson and Howard, 1980.

Fig. 3. Sequences around the Thiolester Sites of C3 (23), C4 (22,24)
and α₂M. (25).

native proteins. In addition, the bond split during autolytic cleavage, a property of the thiolester-containing proteins and requiring
an intact thiolester, is that between glu-25 and glu-26 (27). The
conserved nature of the thiolester site is further illustrated in
Figure 4. The flanking proline residues, together with the hydrophobic
sequences on either side of the site, would stabilise a thiolester
in the native protein. Positions at which there are notable differences in the chemical nature of the amino acids contained in the
three proteins are boxed. These, particularly those amino-terminal
to the thiolester site (e.g. the basic residues in C4), might be involved in determining acceptor specificity.

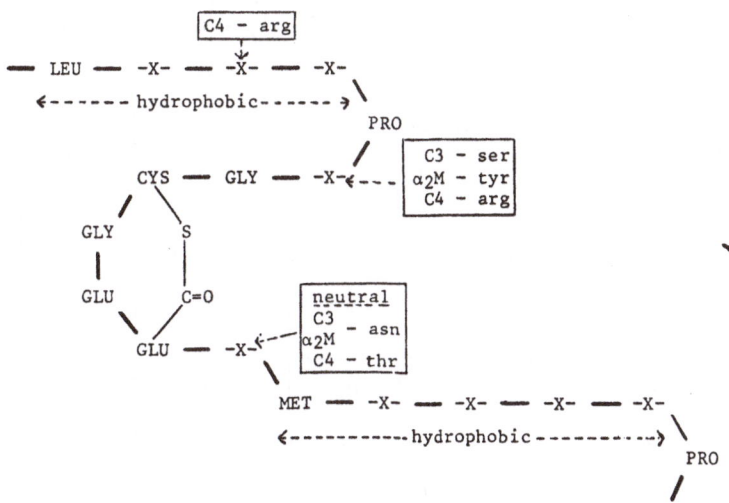

Fig. 4. Structural features around the Thiolester Site

Further Structural and Functional Homologies between Thiolester-Containing Proteins

   While C3, C4 and α_2-macroglobulin show clear sequence homology around the thiolester site, this in itself is not sufficient evidence for a common evolutionary precursor for the three proteins. A common genetic element containing the coding sequence for the thiolester region could, during evolution, have been inserted into otherwise unrelated genes. However the three proteins do have further clear functional similarities. All are activated by a limited proteolytic cleavage, all are capable of forming covalent complexes on activation, and the complexes formed are cleared from the circulation via receptors specific for the activated protein. Further structural and functional comparisons are shown in Table 1. C5, while it does not contain an internal thiolester (12,18), is included as it has long been regarded as being related to C3 and C4, and the activation peptides C3a, C4a, and C5a, now totally sequenced, show a high degree of homology (28).

   C3, C4 and C5 are all synthesised as single chain precursor proteins (29-32). In the case of C3 and C4, the β chain is known to be amino-terminal (33-36). If the amino-terminal sequences of the β chains of C3 and C4 are aligned with that of α_2-macroglobulin (that of C5 has not yet been determined), as shown in Figure 5, limited homology becomes apparent. As was mentioned above, this homology extends through the activation peptides (20% overall homology over 75-80 residues). The next point at which sequence comparison can be made is around the peptide bonds split during activation (Figure 6).

Table 1. Specific Functional and Structural Properties of the Thiolester-Containing Proteins C3, C4, and α_2-macroglobulin, and of the Structurally-Related Protein, C5

	Proteolytic Activation	Activation Peptide	Thiolester	Specific Receptor	Non-Specific Surface Uptake	Cofactor Binding	Factor I Sensitive
α_2M	YES (endoproteases)	NO	YES	YES	(NO)	NO	NO
C3	YES (C4b2a, C3bBb, endoproteases)	YES (C3a)	YES	YES	YES	YES (factor B)	YES (factor H)
C4	YES (C1, endoproteases?)	YES (C4a)	YES	YES	YES	YES (C2)	YES (C4b.p.)
C5	YES (C4b2a3b, C3b$_n$Bb)	YES (C5a)	NO	(YES)	YES	YES (C6)	NO

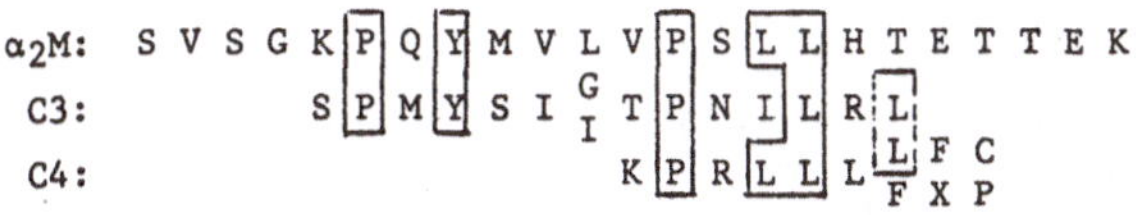

```
α₂M:   S  V  S  G  K P Q Y M  V  L  V P S L L  H  T  E  T  T  E  K
C3:                S P M Y S  I G T P N  I  L R L
                               I                 L F C
C4:                      K P R L L L    F X P
```

α₂M - Sottrup-Jensen et al, 1981.
C3 - Tack et al, 1979; Davis and Harrison, 1982.
C4 - Bolotin et al, 1977; Gigli et al, 1977.

Fig. 5.   Amino-Terminal Sequences of the C3 (37,38) and C4 (39,40)
β Chains and of α₂-Macroglobulin (41).

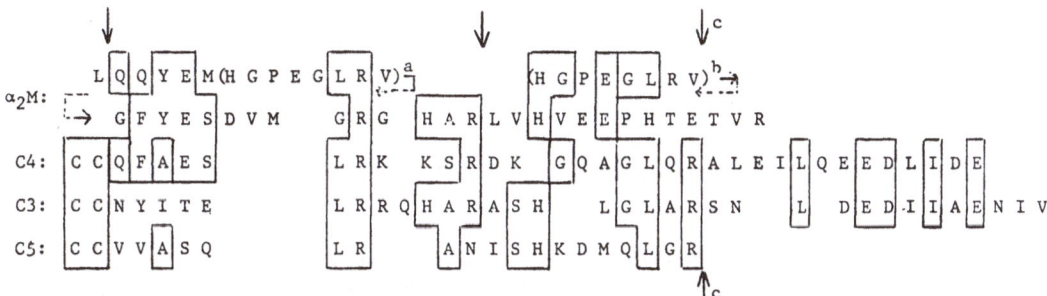

a,b - Alternative alignments of the α₂-macroglobulin sequence suggesting internal homology.
Arrows indicate proteolytic cleavage points, c - physiological cleavage points.

α₂M - Sottrup-Jensen et al, 1981.
C4 - Moon et al, 1981; Press and Gagnon, 1981.
C3 - Hugli, 1975; Tack et al, 1979; Davis and Harrison, 1982.
C5 - Fernandez and Hugli, 1978.

Fig. 6.   Amino Acid Sequences around the Activation Sites of
C3 (37,38,42), C4 (43,44), C5 (28) and α₂-Macroglobulin (41).
a,b - Alternative alignments of the α₂-macroglobulin sequ-
ence suggesting internal homology. Arrows indicate proteo-
lytic cleavage points, c - physiological cleavage points.

Again, sequence homology between α₂-macroglobulin and the carboxy-
terminal regions of the activation peptides is apparent and, in the
case of C3 and C4, homology into the α' chains of C3b and C4b also
exists. (The corresponding sequences for C5 and α₂-macroglobulin have
not yet been determined.) In addition there is a suggestion that
there is internal homology in α₂-macroglobulin, either with the
alignment suggested by Sottrup-Jensen and coworkers (41) (a), or
with that preferred here (b) with the major cleavage points of all
four proteins aligned. It should be noted that although the complement
proteins are activated physiologically at the points indicated (c),
the regions amino-terminal to these, particularly in the case of C3,
are, as with α₂-macroglobulin, susceptible to attack by a large number

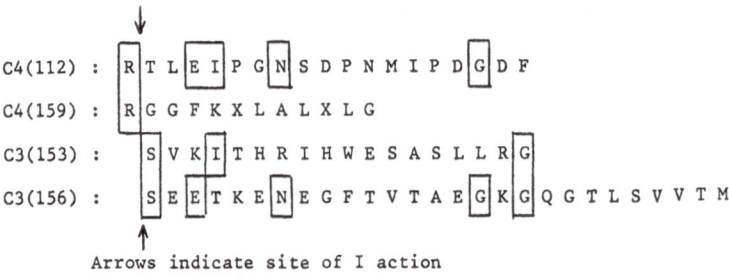

Arrows indicate site of I action

Factor I requires Factor H to act on C3b
                   C4 binding protein to act on C4b

C4 - Press and Gagnon, 1981; C3 - Davis and Harrison, 1982.

Fig. 7. Amino Acid Sequences at the Factor I Cleavage Sites of C4
         and C3 (38,44).

of proteases. The only other point at which sequence comparison can
be made is around the Factor I-mediated cleavage sites of C3 and C4
(Figure 7). Here there is a suprising lack of homology. This point
is emphasised if the precursor complement proteins and α_2-macroglo-
bulin are aligned as in Figure 8. All of the functionally analogous
regions align well linearly, and, with the exception of the Factor I
cleavage sites, show considerable sequence homology. Further consideration of Factor I cleavage of C3b and C4b suggests one possible
explanation for this. Only one of the Factor I cleavage sites in C4,
C4(159), aligns with the Factor H-dependent sites in C3, C3(153) and
C3(156). The other, C4(112), aligns with the recently described
C3(113) cleavage site (45) and a proteolytically labile site in C5,
C5(115) (37,46,47). Neither of these latter sites has been sequenced,
but the C3(113) site is known to require a cofactor other than Factor
H, possibly the CR1 receptor (48,49). In contrast, Factor I action
on C4b requires C4 binding protein. Sequence homology, other than
for absolute structural requirements for Factor I cleavage, would
only be expected between sites that can be aligned (either C3(153)
or C3(156) and C4(159). Lack of homology can be explained in two
ways. Possibly there is no selective pressure on this region other
than to retain a minimum specificity site for Factor I cleavage.
This could be as little as a basic residue (e.g. arginine) on the
amino-terminal side of the site and a small residue (e.g. serine,
glycine or alanine) on the carboxy-terminal side. Higher specificity
would therefore be determined by cofactor binding, the cofactor di-
recting or permitting the proteolytic action. Alternatively the ancestral relationship between the proteins might cease to exist at
some point between the thiolester site and the site of Factor I
action at around 150-160 kilodalton. This second hypothesis is less
attractive because of the close correlation in overall polypeptide
chain length in the four proteins. Sequence information around the
cleavage sites at 112-113 kilodaltons as well as through the carboxy-

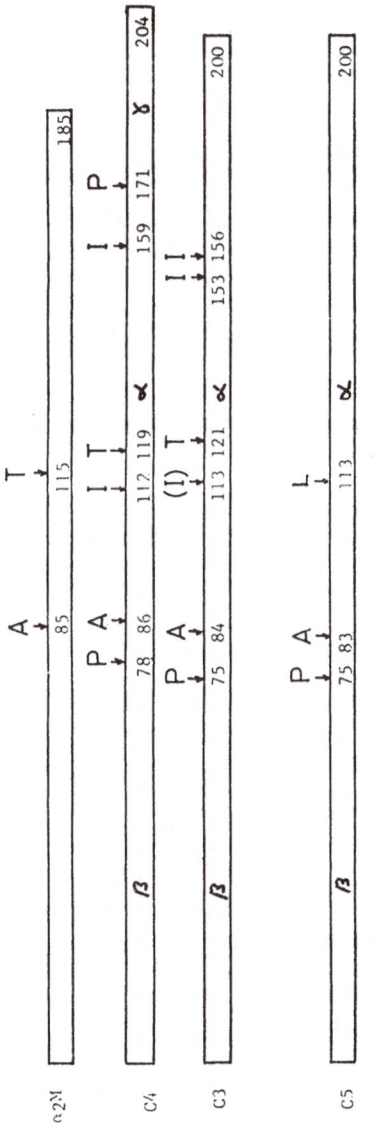

P – Sites of proteolytic cleavage generating functional proteins from single chain
    precursors.

A – Site of proteolytic activation.

T – Thiolester site.

I – Sites of factor I action.

L – Possible position of the proteolytically labile site C5.

Numbers refer to distance in kilodaltons from the amino-termini of the (precursor) polypeptide chains

Fig. 8. Comparison of the Polypeptide Chain Structures of C3, C4, C5 and α_2-Macroglobulin

terminal regions of the polypeptides would be helpful in assessing
these alternatives.

An Evolutionary Scheme for Plasma Thiolester-Containing Proteins

A possible evolutionary pathway for the known thiolester-containing plasma proteins is given in Figure 9. While there is no compel-
ling basis for ascribing a function to the precursor or ancestral
protein (e.g. "protease inhibitor-like" or "complement-like"), the
assumption made here is that it was "complement-like". Indeed, as
has been suggested by Lachmann (50) it might well have possessed
functions that have been retained in C3. However, whatever its role
it would have been highly inefficient compared with the plasma proteins seen today. Possible properties of this protein are summarised
in figure 10. Early divergence of α_2-macroglobulin and the complement
proteins is indicated by the presence of the $\beta-\alpha$ split in the latter
and its absence in the former. Subsequent to this, α_2-macroglobulin
has evolved to become a highly efficient non-specific "protease-
trapping" protease inhibitor, capable of forming a covalent bond with
the protease that activates it. Loss of specificity of activation
might well have been consequent on an internal duplication of the
activation region. At some point, possibly prior to the divergence
of α_2-macroglobulin and the complement proteins, it is possible that
a binding site for the activating protease was aquired, and that with
the complement proteins this became the ancestral proteolytic cofactor. (Certainly it seems likely that parallel evolution of the complement components C3, C4 and C5 and their respective cofactors,
Factor B, C2 and C6, has occurred. This clearly requires closely associated gene duplications of the precursor membrane-binding component and cofactor protease.) Confinement of this site to the surface-
bound protein, together with a significant rate of decay of the complex and inefficient circulation would allow continued but diffusion-
limited expression of proteolytic activity against further complement
protein and therefore a limited amplification of deposition on an
activating particle. In addition, the complement precursor, by virtue
of the $\beta-\alpha$ scission, could release a small peptide (the "a" fragment)
on activation, which, during evolution, aquired a chemotactic activity and hence ability to recruit motile cells to the site of complement deposition. In spite of the closer similarity in terms of polypeptide structure between C3 and C5, and a higher degree of sequence
homology in the "a" fragments (C3a/C5a, 38% homology; C3a/C4a, 30%;
C4a/C5a, 35%), it is likely that C5 diverged from a common C3/C4
precursor. There are three reasons for believing this. Firstly, C5
no longer possesses an internal thiolester (12,51). Secondly, its
cofactor, C6, no longer appears to express proteolytic activity
(although in this context the recent report that C6 reacts with
serine protease-specific reagents should be borne in mind (52).
Certainly C56 does not act proteolytically on the late components
of the lytic pathway. Finally, C3b and C4b, but not C5b, are cleaved,
in the presence of a cofactor, by Factor I. Acquisition of this re-

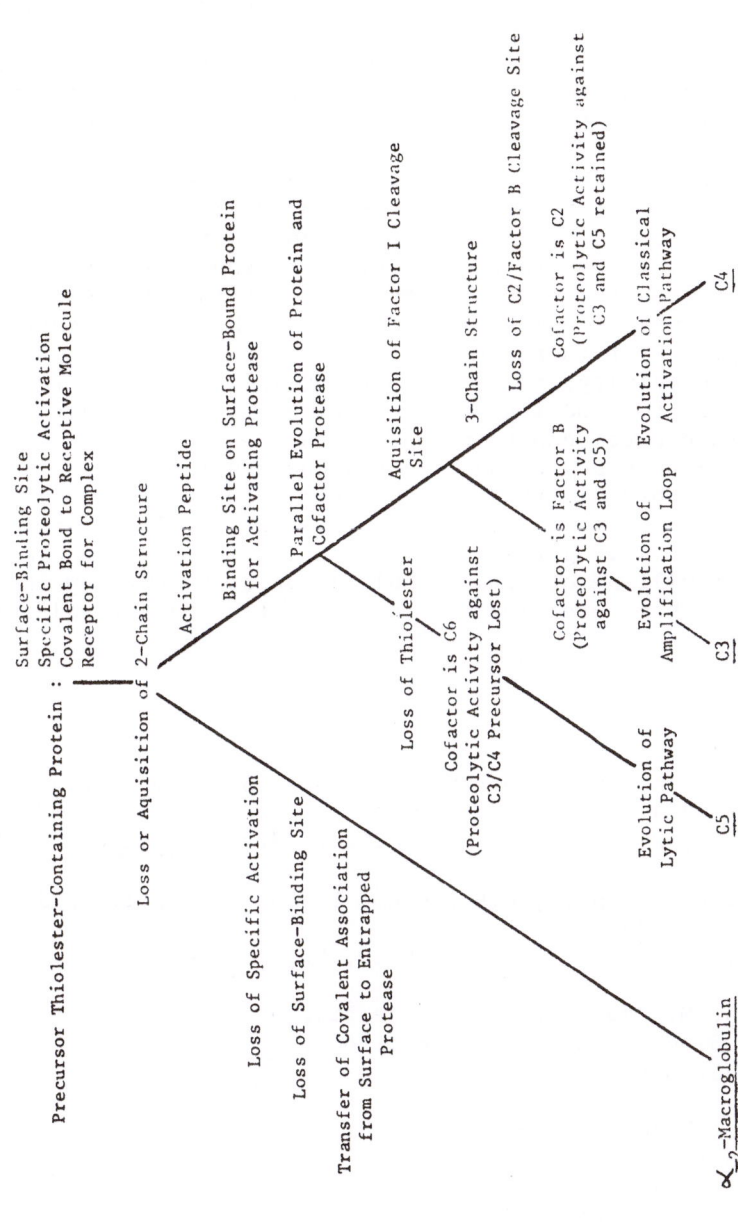

Fig. 9. A Possible Evolutionary Pathway for Plasma Thiolester-Containing Proteins.

gulated expression of proteolytic activity would have permitted,
following further gene duplication, the development of the highly
efficient amplification loop of the alternative pathway and the
linked expression of antigen-antibody interaction and complement activation via the classical pathway. Since there is no apparent requirement for regulation of classical pathway activation at the C42
level, it is possible that in C4 the Factor I cleavage sites are retained as an evolutionary relic.

In this presentation I have outlined the evidence for a common
evolutionary precursor for the three known thiolester-containing
plasma proteins C3, C4 and α_2-macroglobulin and the related complement protein, C5. These are all relatively abundant plasma proteins.
The question arises as to whether there are further members of this
family of proteins. As has been mentioned, we have preliminary evidence to suggest that there are other plasma proteins with a "thio-
lester-like" reactivity, and therefore possible additions to this
family. However, the model-building studies cited earlier showed that
an internal thiolester can be formed in the sequence cys-x-y-glu
where x and y can be any amino acid residue other than proline (23).
It is therefore possible that the absolute structural requirements
for the thiolester site, as yet not understood, could exist in non-
related proteins, giving rise to distinct families with a common
reactivity. It will be of considerable interest to see how our understanding of these proteins and their relationships develop in the
next few years.

REFERENCES

1. Gordon, J., Whitehead, H.R. and Wormall, A., Biochem. J.
    20:1028 (1926).
2. Ecker, E.E., Pillemer, C. and Seifter, S., J. Immunol. 47:181
    (1943).
3. Pillemer, L., Ratnoff, Ρ.D., Blum, L. and Lepow, I.H., J. Exp.
    Med. 97:573 (1953).
4. Pillemer, L., Lepow, I.H. and Blum, L., J. Immunol. 71:339
    (1953).
5. Steinbuch, M., Pejaudier, L,, Quentin, M. and Martin, V.,
    Biochem. Biophys. Acta 154:228 (1968).
6. Müller-Eberhard, H.J. and Gotze, O., J. Exp. Med. 135:1003
    (1972).
7. Müller-Eberhard H.J. and Biro, C.E., J. Exp. Med. 118:447 (1963).
8. Steinbuch, M., Audran, R., Lambin, P. and Fine, J.M., in:
    "Protides of Biological Fluids", ed. H. Peters, p. 133
    Elsevier, Amsterdam (1975).
9. Harpel, P.C., Fed. Proc. 34:344 (1975).
10. Laskowski, M. and Kato, I., Ann. Review Biochem. 49:493 (1980).
11. Law, S.K. and Levine, R.P., Proc. Natl. Acad. Sci. U.S.A.
    74:2701 (1977).

12. Law, S.K., Lichtenberg, N.A., Holcombe, F.H. and Levine, R.P., J. Immunol. 125:634 (1980).
13. Campbell, R.D., Dodds, A.W. and Porter, R.R., Biochem. J. 189:67 (1980).
14. Gadd, K.J. and Reid, K.B.M., Biochem. J. 195:471 (1981).
15. Seifter, S., Katchalski, E. and Harkness, D.M., Fed. Proc. 22:612 (1963).
16. Law, S.K., Lichtenberg, N.A. and Levine, R.P., J. Immunol. 123:1388 (1979).
17. Swenson, R.P. and Howard, J.B., Proc. Natl. Acad. Sci. U.S.A. 76:4313 (1979).
18. Janatova, J., Lorenz, P.E., Schechter, A.N., Prahl, J.W. and Tack, B.F., Biochemistry 19:4471 (1980).
19. Salvesen, G.S. and Barrett, A.J., Biochem. J. 187:695 (1980).
20. Salvesen, G.S., Sayers, C.A. and Barrett, A.J., Biochem. J. 195:453 (1981).
21. Tack, B.F., Harrison, R.A., Janatova, J., Thomas, M.L. and Prahl, J.W., Proc. Natl. Acad. Sci. U.S.A. 77:5764 (1980).
22. Harrison, R.A., Thomas, M.L. and Tack, B.F., Proc. Natl. Acad. Sci. U.S.A. 78:7388 (1981).
23. Thomas, M.L., Janatova, J., Gray, W. and Tack B.F., Proc. Natl. Acad. Sci. U.S.A. 79:1054 (1982).
24. Campbell, R.D., Gagnon, J. and Porter, R.R., Biosciences Reports 1:423 (1981).
25. Swenson, R.P. and Howard, J.B., J. Biol. Chem. 255:8087 (1980).
26. Tack, B.F., Janatova, J., Thomas, M.L. Harrison, R.A. and Hammer, C., in: "Methods in Enzymology", volume 80 (Proteolytic Enzymes, Part C), L. Lorand, ed., p. 64 (1981).
27. Howard, J.B., Vermeulen, M. and Swenson, R.P., J. Biol. Chem. 255:3820 (1980).
28. Fernandez, H.N. and Hugli, T.E., J. Biol. Chem. 253:6955 (1978).
29. Hall, R.E. and Colten, H.R., Proc. Natl. Acad. Sci. U.S.A. 74:1707 (1977).
30. Brade, V., Hall, R.E. and Colten, H.R., J. Exp. Med. 146:759 (1977).
31. Ooi, Y.M. and Colten, H.R., J. Immunol. 123:2494 (1979).
32. Patel, F. and Minta, J.O., J. Immunol. 123:2408 (1979).
33. Goldberger, G., Abraham, G.N., Williams, J. and Colten, H.R., J. Biol. Chem. 255:7071 (1980).
34. Parker, K.L., Schreffier, D.C. and Capra, J.D., Proc. Natl. Acad. Sci. U.S.A. 77:4275 (1980).
35. Sim, R.B. and Sim, E., Biochem. J. 193:129 (1981).
36. Goldberger, G., Thomas, M.L., Tack, B.F., Williams, J., Colten, H.R. and Abrahams, G.N., J. Biol. Chem. 256:12617 (1981).
37. Tack, B.F., Morris, S.C. and Prahl, J.W., Biochemistry 18:1490 (1979).
38. Davis, A.E. and Harrison, R.A., Biochemistry (in the press), (1982).
39. Bolotin, C., Morris, S.C., Tack, B.F. and Prahl, J.W., Biochemistry 16:2008 (1977).

40. Gigli, I., von Zabern, I. and Porter, R.R., <u>Biochem. J.</u> 165:439 (1977).
41. Sottrup-Jensen, L., Lonblad, P.B., Stepanik, T.M., Petersen, T.E., Magnusson, S. and Jornvall, P., <u>F.E.B.S. Lett.</u> 127:167 (1981).
42. Hugli, T.E., J. <u>Biol. Chem.</u> 250:8293 (1975).
43. Moon, K.E., Gorski, J.P. and Hugli, T.E., <u>J. Biol. Chem.</u> 256:8685 (1981).
44. Press, E.M. and Gagnon, J., <u>Biochem. J.</u> 199:351 (1981).
45. Medicus, R.M. and Arnaout, A., <u>Molec. Immunol.</u> (in press) (1982).
46. Nilsson, U.R., Mandle, R.J. and McConnell-Mapes, J.A., <u>J. Immunol.</u> 114:815 (1975).
47. Yamamoto, K,I. and Gewurz, H., <u>J. Immunol.</u> 120:2008 (1978).
48. Ross, G.D., Lambris, J.D., Cain, J.A. and Newman, S.L., <u>J. Immunol.</u> (in press), (1982).
49. Medof, M.E., Iida, K., Mold, C. and Nussenzweig, V., <u>J. Exp. Med.</u> (in press), (1982).
50. Lachmann, P.J., <u>Behring Inst. Mitt.</u> 63:25 (1979).
51. Janatova, J. and Tack, B.F., <u>Biochemistry</u> 20:2394 (1981).
52. Kolb, W.P., Kolb, L.M. and Savary, J.R., <u>Biochemistry</u> 21:294 (1982).

STRUCTURAL ANALYSIS OF CLONED MOUSE AND HUMAN DNA SEQUENCES
SPECIFYING C3, THE THIRD COMPONENT OF COMPLEMENT

G. Fey, K. Wiebauer, H. Domdey, M. Kazmaier,
C. Southgate and V. Müller

Department of Molecular Biology
Swiss Institute for Experimental Cancer Research
CH 1066 Epalinges, Switzerland

INTRODUCTION

We wished to produce cloned DNA sequences representing C3, the
third component of complement and to perform structural characterization of these for three principal purposes. Firstly, we wanted to
predict the primary amino acid sequences of the C3 polypeptide from
nucleotide sequences of cloned complementary DNA (cDNA). The C3 protein possesses multiple functions due to its capacity to interact
specifically with other complement components (e.g. convertase complexes in the classical and alternative pathway), the control proteins I and H of the alternative pathway of complement activation
and with several different types of C3 receptor molecules in the
surface membranes of different classes of cells (1-4). Inspite of
the important role of C3 in the defence of the human organism against
infection and inspite of the fact, that it can be purified in large
quantities (5), only very scarce primary amino acid sequence data
have been accumulated. The published sequences cover: the C3a anaphylatoxin peptide (6,7), the amino- and carboxy- termini of the mature
α, α' and β subunits (8,9), the aminoterminus of the pro-C3 precursor polypeptide (10) and the part of the C3d peptide fragment, that
contains the internal thiolester site (11,12). The large size of the
C3 polypeptide (approx. Mol Wt 190 000) may have discouraged investigators from tempting to determine its complete amino acid sequence.
It is possible to predict amino acid sequence from nucleotide sequences of cloned cDNA, and such data together with protein sequence
data from selected regions of the polypeptide are expected to produce
the complete primary structure of this important protein. The next
important task after establishing the primary sequence will be to
map the various ligand interacting sites on the C3 polypeptide chain.

For this purpose cloned cDNA may also be useful, because it may allow to produce wild-type and mutated peptide fragments in bacteria
and to measure their functional capacities. Cloned genomic DNA may
become useful to delineate functionally important domains of the
polypeptide by transfection/transformation studies with wild-type
and altered DNA sequences. Secondly, we want to analyze the over all
exon-intron block structure of the gene and to generate restriction
enzyme cleavage maps of it. Knowledge of the structural organization
of a wild-type copy of the gene will provide the basis for future
characterization of inherited human C3 deficiency alleles (13-15).
Thirdly, we would like to study control mechanisms, that govern the
expression of the C3 gene into RNA and protein. This gene is subjected to several known controls: (a) it is expressed in a clearly
tissue-specific manner, liver hepatocytes are the principal site of
synthesis (reviewed in ref. 16) and extrahepatic synthesis occurs
mainly in cells of the macrophage/monocyte series (17) and to a les-
ser extent in gut associated epithelial cells (18) and in skin fibro-
blasts (19), but it is not expressed in most other tissues., (b) it
is expressed with increased rates of synthesis during acute inflammation (20) and (c) it can be regulated by steroid hormones (21,22).
We would like to use cloned DNA sequences as tools to titrate the
production of C3 RNA-species in various tissues and their increased
synthesis under the influence of a variety of stimulating agents
such as inflammatory substances and glucocorticoid hormones.

RESULTS AND DISCUSSION

    I. Mouse C3 cDNA. Mouse C3 cDNA was produced by reverse trans-
cription of a high molecular weight size fraction (longer than 5 000
nucleotides) of mouse liver messenger RNA (mRNA), inserted into the
plasmid vector pBR 322 and cloned in E.coli using standard technology (23). A series of eight different recombinant cDNA plasmids
(clones) with partially overlapping inserts were obtained, and a
restriction enzyme cleavage map was established. The size of mouse
C3 mRNA was measured to be 5 100 ± 200 nucleotides, including a poly
A-tail with mean length of 170 adenosine nucleotides (24). The
cloned cDNA sequence represent 4 700 nucleotides of the 5 100 nucleotide mRNA, including its 3' end. The extreme 5' end of the mRNA was
not represented by cloned cDNA, but genomic DNA clones covering this
region are available. Partial DNA sequence analysis was performed
on selected cDNA regions and five main elements of information could
be derived:

a. The amino acid sequence of the mouse C3a anaphylatoxin peptide
    and some flanking amino acid sequences in the precursor pro-C3
    molecule were derived. Mouse C3a is homologous with rat C3a in
    72 out of 78 amino acid residues and with human and porcine C3a
    in 52 and 50 respectively out of 77 residues. Thus, the cDNA
    sequence predicts extensive homology between the anaphylatoxin

peptides of mice and other species.

b. The order of subunits in the precursor pro-C3 molecule could be
    established to be: NH_2 -β- α-COOH, confirming results of others
    (10).

c. The cDNA sequence predicts that in the transition region between
    the carboxyterminus of the β-chain and the aminoterminus of the
    α-chain, four arginine residues should be contained in pro-C3,
    which should not appear in the mature β- and α-subunits, and
    which should be removed during the processing steps from the
    precursor to the mature subunits.

d. cDNA sequences imply that the initial translation product from
    C3 mRNA should be pre-pro-C3 molecule, carrying an aminoterminal
    extension peptide. This so-called signal- or leader-peptide has
    been sequenced on the level of genomic DNA (see below).

e. The sequence containing the internal thiolester site in the C3d
    region is predicted to be: Gly-Cys-Gly-Glu-GlN-AsN-Met in good
    homology with the corresponding sequence in the human C3 protein
    (homology in 6/7 residues, ref. 11,12). Unexpectedly, residue 5
    in this sequence, which participates in the thiolester bond, is
    predicted to be encoded as a glutamine. When the human protein
    was sequenced after hydrolysis of the bond, this residue appeared
    as a glutamic acid (11,12). The sequence suggests, that the glu-
    tamic acid may be the result of a posttranslational modification.

II. The Mouse C3 Gene. A gene library of liver DNA from strain
A mice was constructed in the phage replacement vector lambda 1059
and by screening with radiolabelled cloned cDNA probes, four recombinant phages were isolated. Together their inserts contain one full
copy of a mouse C3 gene (25). The inserts of two of these phages
span a strech of 32 kilobasepairs (kb) of mouse DNA, containing
24 kb of the gene and 1.2 kb of 5'- and 7 kb of 3'- flanking sequences. The 5'- and 3'- ends of the gene were precisely mapped and
restriction enzyme cleavage maps for the enzymes Bam HI, HindIII
and EcoRI were established. A fragment of 240 nucleotides containing
the 5' end of the gene was sequenced. A so-called TATA-box, a sequence element signalling and RNA-polymerase II promoter region, was
found and the 5' end of the mRNA (cap-site) was mapped. The AUG
translation initiation codon was found after a 56 nucleotide 5' non-
translated region of the mRNA. The genomic DNA then contains coding
sequences for a 24 amino acid residue signal- or leader-peptide of
typical amino acid composition and sequence. This signal peptide
and the next two amino acids are encoded by a separate first exon
of the gene (25). Comparative Southern-blot hybridizations were performed using liver DNA from strain A mice and DNA from a mixture of
the two recombinant phages that span the entire gene. The pattern

of restriction enzyme fragments generated by digestion of genomic
DNA with the enzymes Bam HI, HindIII and EcoRI was indistinguishable
from the corresponding patterns obtained with DNA from the recombinant phages. The interpretation is, that the mouse genome contains
only one type of C3 gene. One can not conclude from this result,
that it would contain only one copy of the gene per haploid set of
chromosomes. The copy number still needs to be titrated by quantitative nucleic acid hybridization experiments. However, it appears,
that the C3 gene is not a member of a small gene family, which would
contain other related but variant genes. In particular, no evidence
for the existence of so-called pseudogenes has been obtained. Such
functionally inactive gene copies have frequently been observed for
other genes. The mouse C3 gene behaves as a strict single copy gene.
If the genome contains more than one copy per haploid amount of DNA,
then all these copies should give rise to indistinguishable Bam HI,
EcoRI and HindIII restriction patterns. While this is not excluded,
it appears unlikely, because one would expect rapid divergence of
intron sequences, and thus of the restriction patterns, between the
various copies of the gene.

    III. The Human C3 Gene. In Southern blot experiments with paral-
lel samples of mouse and human genomic DNA it was observed, that
radiolabelled mouse C3 cDNA probes crosshybridized extensively with
a variety of restriction fragments of the human C3 gene (K. Wiebauer
and G. Fey, unpublished data). Therefore the sequence homology between the two genes seems not to be confined to a few restricted
regions, but rather to be spread over an extended portion of both
genes. Consequently mouse cDNA probes could be used to identify
cloned human C3 DNA sequences. A human genomic DNA library contained
on lambda phage vectors was kindly provided to us by Dr. Tom
Maniatis, Harvard University, and was screened with radiolabelled
mouse C3 cDNA probes. One recombinant phage, lambda HuC3 RI No. 5
was isolated. It contains a 17 kb insert of human DNA consisting of
two neighboring 5 and 12 kb EcoRI fragments of the human C3 gene.
In Southern blot experiments with DNA samples from seven unrelated
human individuals the 12 kb band was always seen, whereas the 5 kb
fragment was not. Therefore we have subcloned a unique-sequence
(non-repetitive) 1.39 kb pstI fragment from the 12 kb EcoRI fragment on the plasmid vector pxf3 and on the M 13 phage mp7. The
recombinant plasmid pxHuC3 1.39/132 hybridizes to coding sequences
from the central portion of the mouse C3 alpha chain and represents
our best probe for human C3 sequences, while human C3 cDNA clones
are not yet available. With the help of this probe, the human C3
gene was mapped on human chromosome 19 using DNA from a panel of
mouse-human somatic-cell hybrids that contained only restricted
subsets of human chromosomes (26). This probe has recently also been
used by other laboratories to map other genes in the vicinity of
the human C3 gene on chromosome 19. Linkage studies were performed
between recognizable alleles of these other genes and polymorphic

alleles of the C3 gene, recognizable with these probes by their polymorphic restriction enzyme cleavage patterns in Southern blot experiments (Drs. K.E. Davies and H.H. Ropers, personal communication).

A human gene library (the J.G. library) constructed on the cosmid vector pTM was kindly provided to us by Drs. F. Grosveld and R. Flavell from Mill Hill, England. This library was screened with the 1.39 kb fragment cloned in phage M13 mp7 as a probe and three recombinant cosmids were isolated, which contain overlapping inserts of 28,34 and 36 kb. These inserts must represent overlapping portions of the human C3 gene, because they all hybridize with this probe. Present efforts aim at the mapping of the 5' and 3' ends of the gene and at the preparation of restriction enzyme cleavage maps for these cosmid inserts. It is expected that these clones will provide valuable starting material for the characterization of the wild type human C3 gene and a basis for future studies of inherited human C3 deficiency alleles and of the control of expression of the C3 gene.

Acknowledgments

This work was supported by a research grant from the Swiss National Science Foundation. K. Wiebauer and H. Domdey were recipients of postdoctoral fellowships by EMBO and DFG (Deutsche Forschungs Gemeinschaft). C. Southgate was awarded a student fellowship from the Swiss Cancer Research Institute.

We thank Drs. T. Maniatis, F. Grosveld and R. Flavell for the human gene libraries and gifts of placenta tissue and DNA. We are indebted to Drs. B. Hirt and H. Diggelmann for support and to our colleagues Drs. U. Schibler, O. Hagenbuechle, P. Wellauer, S. Bodary, N. Fasel and R. Sahli for stimulating discussions.

REFERENCES

1. Müller-Eberhard, H.J. and Schreiber, R.D., Adv. Immunol. 29:1-53 (1980).
2. Reid, K.B.M. and Porter, R.R., Ann. Rev. Biochem. 50:433-464 (1981).
3. Fearon, D.T., J. Exp. Med. 152:20-30 (1980).
4. Lambris, J.D., Dobson, N.J. and Ross, G.D., Proc. Natl. Acad. Sci. USA 78:1828-1832 (1981).
5. Hammer, C.H., Wirtz, G.H., Renfer, L., Gresham, H.D. and Tack, B.F., J. Biol. Chem. 256:3995-4006 (1981).
6. Hugli, T.E. and Müller-Eberhard, H.J., Adv. Immunol. 26:1-53 (1979).
7. Hugli, T.E., CRC Critic. Rev. Immunol. 1:321-366 (1981).
8. Tack, B.F., Morris, S.C. and Prahl, J.W., Biochemistry

18:1497–1503 (1979).

9. Thomas, M.L. and Tack, B.F., Biochemistry (1982) (in press).
10. Goldberger, G., Thomas, M.L., Tack, B.F., Williams, J., Colten, H.R. and Abraham, G.N., J. Biol. Chem. 256:12617–12619 (1981).
11. Thomas, M.L., Janatova, J., Gray, W.R. and Tack, B.F., Proc. Natl. Acad. Sci. USA 79:1054–1058 (1982).
12. Campbell, R.D., Gagnon, J. and Porter, R.R., Biochem. J. 199:359–370 (1981).
13. Alper, C.A., Colten, H.R., Rosen, F.S., Rabson, A.R., Macnab, G.M. and Gear, J.S.S., Lancet 2:1179–1181 (1972).
14. Einstein, L.P., Hansen, P.J., Ballow, M., Davies, A.E.III, Danis, J.S.IV., Alper, C.A., Rosen, F.S. and Colten, H.R., J. Clin. Invest. 60:963–969 (1977).
15. Roord, J.J., Daha, M., Kuis, W., Verbrugh, H.A., Verhoef, J., Zegers, B.J.M. and Stoop, J.W., (1982) (in press).
16. Alper, C.A. and Nathan, D.G., in: "Hematology of Infancy and Childhood", (Eds. D.G., Nathan and F.A., Oski), pp. 1459–1490, W.B. Saunders, Philadelphia, (1981).
17. Colten, H.R., Ooi, Y.M. and Edelson, P.J., Ann. N. Y. Acad. Sci. 332:482–490 (1979).
18. Fey, G. and Colten, H.R., Fed. Proc. Fedn. Am. Socs. Exp. Biol. 40:2099–2104 (1981).
19. Whitehead, A.S., Sim, R.B. and Bodmer, W.F., Eur. J. Immunol. 11:140–146 (1981).
20. Kushner, I., Edgington, T.S., Trimble, C., Liem, H.H. and Müller-Eberhard, U., J. Lab. Clin. Med. 80:18–25 (1972).
21. Propp, R.P. and Alper, C.A., Science 162:672–673 (1968).
22. Strunk, R.C., Tashjian, A.H. and Colten, H.R., J. Immunol. 114:331–335 (1975).
23. Odink, K.G., Fey, G., Wiebauer, K. and Diggelmann, H., J. Biol. Chem. 256:1453–1458 (1981).
24. Domdey, H., Wiebauer, K., Kazmaier, M., Müller, V., Odink, K. and Fey, G., Proc. Natl. Acad. Sci. USA (1982) (in press).
25. Wiebauer, K., Domdey, H., Diggelmann, H. and Fey, G., Proc. Natl. Acad. Sci. USA (1982) (in press).
26. Whitehead, A.S., Solomon, E., Chambers, S., Bodmer, W.F., Povey, S. and Fey, G., Proc. Natl. Acad. Sci. USA 79:5021–5025 (1982).

HLA ENCODED GENES AND THEIR ASSOCIATIONS WITH DISEASE

G. Hauptmann

Institut d'Hématologie and Centre de Transfusion
Sanguine, Strasbourg, France

The relatively recent discovery concerning the situation of
the structural loci for three major complement proteins: Factor B,
C2 and C4 in the Major Histocompatibility Complex (MHC) gives a new
dimension to this complex. The reasons for this association are
still not clear but practical use has been made of the close linkage
and the resulting linkage disequilibrium with the MHC genes for the
exploration of the genetic control of the immune response and of the
etiology and pathogeny of some HLA-associated diseases.

Genetics of Factor B (BF), C2 and C4

In man, four complement genes are associated with the HLA
genes:

One gene for Factor B with two common (F,S), two less common
(F1, S0.7 or S1) and several rare genes. The existence of a "null"
or "silent gene" or "QO" (quantitatively zero) gene has not been
definitively proven but one dysfunctional variant (F0.55) has been
described (1).

One gene for C2 with one common allele (C2-C or C2-1), one less
common allele (C2-B or C2-2), two rare alleles (C2-A and C2-A1) and
a "null" gene (C2-QO) responsible for heterozygous or homozygous C2
deficiency.

C4 is controlled by two closely linked loci: C4A (or F) and
C4B (or S). By transposition on the red cells the C4A products give
rise to antigenic determinants described as "Rodgers" for C4A and
"Chido" for C4B (2). "Null" alleles are relatively frequent in this

system either at the A locus or at the B locus but rarely at both
loci together. In general, the products of the C4A locus are hemo-
lytically less active than the products of the C4B locus. One C4A
product, C4A6 is devoid of hemolytical activity.

The polymorphism of Factor B (BF) was first described by Alper
et al. (3) and is generally evidenced by high voltage agarose electrophoresis and immunofixation. Population studies have shown that
the S allele predominates amongst caucasoids, orientals and indians
whereas amongst blacks the F allele predominates. In some mediter-
ranean populations, for instance the Basques, a high frequency of
BF-F1 has been observed (4).

C2 polymorphism was discovered by Hobart and Lachmann (5) and
further studied by Alper et al. (6) and Meo et al. (7) by isoelectric
focusing of serum and hemolytic revelation. Because the C2-C or C2-1
allele is very common, the families informative for C2 are relatively rare. Nevertheless a linkage disequilibrium between C2 and HLA
has been observed. Very interesting is the association of C2-QO and
HLA-B18, DR2, BF-S and C4A4B2. At present, the best markers for C2
deficiency are BF-S, C4A4B2 and HLA-B18 (8).

The definition of the structural polymorphism of C4 has been a
problem because the patterns obtained by electrophoresis and immunofixation are complicated and because the initial attempts to understand this polymorphism assumed the existence of a single C4 locus.
O'Neill et al. showed clearly in 1978 (9) that the bands produced
on electrophoresis in native plasma could not be the products of a
single locus and that there must be two closely linked loci. They
further demonstrated the relationship between C4 types and the so-
called "Chido" and "Rodgers" blood groups. The major problems of the
C4 system were resolved by the introduction of the neuraminidase
treatment of whole plasma before electrophoresis by Awdeh and
Alper (10). By removing sialic acid, a better separation is achieved
of most of the products of the C4A from the C4B loci. With this
technique, at least 8 structural variants at C4A and at least 10 at
C4B could be detected in addition to the "null" gene "QO" at each
locus:
      C4A3 is the common allele at the C4A locus.
      C4B1 is the common allele at the C4B locus.

The relatively high frequency of the "null" genes gives rise
to a high proportion of partial defects of C4 in the general population. About 3 p. cent of individuals are homozygous for BQO, 2 p.
cent are homozygous for AQA and about 5 p. cent are double-
heterozygous BQO and 4QO. In contrast, the occurrence of a C4 "null"
haplotype (AQO and BQO on the same chromosome) is very rare. Individuals homozygous for this haplotype, mainly by consanguinity,
present with a complete C4 deficiency. Only 15 such individuals
have now been disclosed.

The complement genes within HLA

The complement genes associated with the HLA genes are located between HLA-B and HLA-D and represent the genes of the class III, so-called "metabolic genes". These genes are very close together because no recombination has been observed up to now between them and the exact order of the genes is not established but it seems that C4B is closer to HLA-D than C4A. As for the HLA genes there are associations or linkage disequilibrium between C2, C4 and BF genes. Awdeh and Alper have proposed the designation of "complotypes" for these associations. There are also characteristic associations between the "complotypes" and HLA haplotypes and it is now clear that the complement genes allow for a better definition of the haplotypes in linkage disequilibrium. Some well known HLA haplotypes can be completed by the complement markers, for instance:

HLA-A1	Cw7	B8	DR3	with	BF-S	C2-1	C4AQOB1
Aw30	Cw5	B18	DR3	with	BF-F1	C2-1	C4A3BQO
A1	Cw6	B17	DR7	with	BF-S	C2-1	C4A6B1
A25	-	B18	DR2	with	BF-S	C2-QO	C4A4B2
		Bw50		with	BF-SO.7	C2-1	C4A2B1

HLA-complement haplotypes and diseases

Considerable work has been applied in the last years to the associations between diseases and HLA types. One of the problems which recently arose is the question whether the HLA-linked complement genes and their variants could play a role in the etiology or pathogeny of HLA-linked or associated diseases. Precise studies in this field will be difficult because they will need: family studies; typing for HLA-A,B,C,DR; typing for C2, BF and C4; immunochemical and functional titrations of C2, BF, C4 and also of some non-HLA linked complement genes. In fact, relatively few studies including complement markers have been published up to now. However, they indicate that the complement genes could play a role in the occurrence of diseases primarily associated with HLA-D/DR genes such as: insulin-dependent diabetes; multiple sclerosis; lupus erythematosus; idiopathic membranous nephropathy; coeliac disease. All these diseases are related to an abnormal immune response (11).

· Insulin-dependent diabetes: in this disease several susceptibility haplotypes have been identified and one haplotype is thought to protect against the disease:

```
Susceptibility haplotypes: A1  ,Cw7,B8  /BFS, C2C,C4AQOB1/DR3
                           A2  ,Cw3,Bw62/BFS, C2C,C4A3B3 /DR4
                           Aw30,Cw5,B18 /BFF1,C2C,C4A3BQO/DR3
                           A-  ,Cw3,B40 /BFS ,C3C,C4AQOB2/DR4
Protective haplotype     : A3  ,    B7  /BFS, C2C,C4A3B1 /DR2
```

All the susceptibility haplotypes comprise either a C4 "null"
gene AQO or BQO, or variants such as BFF1 or C4B3 which are rare alleles. In contrast, the protective haplotype comprises only common
complement genes.

A high frequency of BFF1 was reported in young diabetics by
several authors. This was particularily true in the French Basque
population (12,13). In this population the haplotype HLA-Aw30,Cw5,
B18/BFF1,C2C,C4A3BQO/DR3 was frequently found in the controls but
much more frequently in the diabetic patients. It could be shown
that:
    Insulin-dependent diabetes is primarily associated with HLA-DR3.
    The disease susceptiblity seems to be influenced by other ge-
netic components of the haplotype.
    C4A3BQO is particularily associated with early onset of the
disease: BQO has a frequency of 87% with age at onset under 20 years
versus 57% in the other patients. The difference is less pronounced
for BFF1 (13). Many patients were homozygous for BQO.

Beside the Basque population, two observations of very early
onset of diabetes in subjects homozygous for C4BQO have been reported (14,15).

Multiple sclerosis: in this disease there is an increase of two
haplotypes: HLA-A3,B7,DR2 with the complement markers BFS,C2C,C4A3B1
          HLA-A1,B8,DR3 with the complement markers BFS,C2C,C4AQOB1

One haplotype comprises a C4 "null" gene AQO. Low levels of C2
have been reported in some patients (16) probably in relation to a
heterozygous C2 deficiency.

Psoriasis vulgaris: the increase of HLA-Cw6 in this disease may
be related to an increase or HLA-B17 and C4A6B1,BFS,C2C. The C4A6
variant is a non functional variant of C4.

Coeliac disease: here again three haplotypes comprising a C4
"null" gene AQO or BQU were found with increased frequency:
          HLA-B18,BFF1,C2C,C4A3BQO,DR3
          HLA-B8 ,BFS ,C2C,C4AQOB1,DR3
          HLA-B12,BFF ,C2C,C4A3BQO,DR7

Lupus erythematosus: this auto-immune disease is sometimes associated with the HLA-A1,B8,BFS,C2C,C4AQOB1,DR3 haplotype.

Idiopathic membranous nephropathy: Dyer et al. (17) reported
on a higher frequency of BFF1 related mainly to HLA-B18,DR3.

IgA nephropathy: Mc Lean et al. (IXth International Complement
Workshop, Key Biscayne, Florida, 1981) observed a higher proportion
of C4BQO homozygotes amongst the patients versus the controls.

Grave's disease: Tom and Farid (18) found reduced levels of C4 in HLA-B8 positive patients versus controls. HLA-B8 individuals are almost always C4AQOB1.

Possible signification of the HLA-complement associations in diseases

The recently reported studies in this field can mainly be considered as preliminary. They indicate that specific complement alleles or "null" genes may contribute to the occurrence of diseases in association with other HLA-linked susceptibility genes.

It seems probable that a linkage disequilibrium between complement genes and HLA genes was maintained because these genes interact in some way and in some situations within the immune response. However, it is not yet established how these genes interact. It is also not established how the different allelic products of C2, C4 and factor B interact together and with the other components of the complement cascade in the expression of the different biological activities derived from the complement activation.

Biological activities related to C2, C4 and factor B are multiple. They concern – activation of macrophages/monocytes
- vasopermeability
- virus neutralization
- immune adherence
- clearance of immune-complexes
- probably normal antibody formation

Therefore the study of the HLA-linked complement genes represents not only a theoretical interest for the multiplication of genetic markers but also includes practical applications and above all raises new very interesting perspectives in research.

REFERENCES

1. Mauff, G., Federmann, G. and Hauptmann, G., Immunobiol. 158:96–100 (1980).
2. O'Neill, G.J., Yang, S.Y., Tegoli, J., Berger, R. and Dupont, B., Nature 273:668–670 (1978).
3. Alper, C.A., Boenisch, T. and Watson, L., J. Exp. Med. 135:68–80 (1972).
4. Ohayon, E., Mouzon, A. De, Hauptmann, G., Klein, J., Abbal, M., Constans, J., Mayer, S. and Ducos, J., J. Immunogenet. 7:441–445 (1980).
5. Hobart, M.J. and Lachmann, P.J., Transplant. Rev. 32:26–42 (1976).
6. Alper, C.A., J. Exp. Med. 144:1111–1115 (1976).

7. Meo, T., Atkinson, J., Bernoco, M., Bernoco, D. and Ceppellini, R., Eur. J. Immunol. 7:916-919 (1976).

8. Hauptmann, G., Tongio, M.M., Goetz, J., Mayer, S., Fauchet, R., Sobel, A., Griscelli, C., Berthoux, F., Rivat, C. and Rother, U., J. Immunogenet. 9:127-132 (1982).

9. O'Neill, G.J., Yang, S.Y. and Dupont, B., Proc. Natl. Acad. Sci. 75:5165-5169 (1978).

10. Awdeh, Z.L. and Alper, C.A., Proc. Nat. Acad. Sci. 77:3576-3580 (1980).

11. Rittner, Ch. and Bertrams, J., Hum. Genet. 56:235-247 (1981).

12. Cambon-de Mouzon, A., Ohayon, E., Ducos, J. and Hauptmann, G., Lancet 2:1364 (1980).

13. Cambon-de Mouzon, A., Ohayon, E., Hauptmann, G., Sevin, A., Abbal, M., Sommer, E., Vergnes, H., Ducos, J., Tissue Antigens 19:366-379 (1982).

14. Champsaur, H.F., Bottazzo, G.F., Bertrams, J., Assan, R. and Bach, Ch. J.Pediat. 100:15-20 (1982).

15. Kurtz, F., Hauptmann, G., Juif, J.G. and Bonardi, J.M., Arch. Franc. Pédiatr. 38:543-545 (1981).

16. Trouillas, P., Berthoux, F., Boisson, D., Aimard, G. and Devic, M., Lancet 2:1023 (1976).

17. Dyer, P.A., Klouda, P.T., Harris, R. and Mallick, N.P., Tissue Antigens 15:505-507 (1980).

18. Tom, W. and Farid, N.R., Hum. Hered. 31:227-231 (1981).

ARTIFICIAL ANTIGENS AND SYNTHETIC VACCINES

A REVIEW

Ruth Arnon

Department of Chemical Immunology
The Weizmann Institute of Science
Rehovot, Israel

SYNTHETIC ANTIGENS

The field of synthetic antigens is a relatively young one in immunology. It started as an isoteric topic, but has developed into a multipronged tool in both basic and applied research.

The advent of synthetic antigens permitted a systematic study concerned with the molecular basis of antigenicity, and allowed better understanding, at a molecular level, of cellular immunological phenomena. Being immunogenic requires some features which depend on more than the molecular parameters of the specific antigenic determinant. The immunogen must be a macromolecule which is foreign to the animal; in many cases, the response to macromolecules is under genetic control. On the other hand, the specificity of molecular recognition between antigen and antibody can be studied with substances which are not immunogenic by themselves, and were termed haptens. These are usually small molecules that when attached to a macromolecular carrier, elicit the formation of antibodies which in turn bind to them.

Is is clear today that even large naturally occurring immunogens (e.g., proteins) are composed of several different antigenic determinants which, when excised from the macromolecule, can be considered haptens. Such haptens or antigenic determinants can be used to study in solution the nature of the antibody combining site by direct binding measurement or by inhibition of the reaction of the antibody with the original antigen. In many cases the antigenic specificity of such determinants, in contrast to small haptens, depends on the conformation of the peptide.

After initial studies demonstrating the capacity of peptides to confer antigenic properties, the research was extended to include dozens of synthetic polymers of amino acids. This synthetic approach offers the advantage that, once the immunogenicity of one synthetic material has been unequivocally demonstrated, many analogs could be prepared and tested. Knowing the chemistry of such copolymers made it possible to arrive at conclusions concerning the role of various structural features in the antigenic functions. Thus it was found that the two most crucial molecular parameters which determine the antigenic properties of synthetic antigens are on the one hand accessibility of the antigenic determinants on the surface of the antigen molecule (so as to be available for recognition by antibodies and the immunocompetent cells) and on the other hand the structural conformation of the antigen.

These two molecular parameters were found to be the decisive factors in determining the immunological properties of natural proteins as well: in all the proteins that have been investigated, the antigenic determinants were located at "corners" or folded regions in the molecular structure, all treatments causing denaturation or loss of folded spatial structure resulted in parallel drastic change of antigenic properties. Utilizing this information it was possible to synthesize an antigenic determinant of a globular protein. The first attempt was made with hen egg white lysozyme. An immunopotent region of the molecule denoted "loop" has been synthesized and attached to a synthetic carrier. Antibodies elicited by immunization with this conjugate reacted with the native lysozyme through a conformation-dependent antigenic determinant. This finding, which was later corroborated by results with other proteins, opened conceptually the road to synthetic vaccines.

Genetic Control of the Immune Response

Immunity is one biological phenomenon which is acquired and can not be inherited. Nevertheless, it is clear today that the capacity to respond well or poorly to a certain antigenic stimulus is under strict genetic control. This observation has been made largely thanks to synthetic antigens, simple chemically, and inbred strains of animals (mice, guinea pigs), simple genetically. Using defined branched synthetic polypeptides differing only in a limited manner within their antigenic determinants, it was possible to prove conclusively that the genetic control of immune response is determinant specific. Thus, one synthetic antigen, denoted (T,G)-A--L let to high antibody response in one strain of mice but to a very low response in another strain. Replacing the tyrosine with histidine led to no response in the first strain of mice and high response in the second. Replacing the tyrosine with phenylalanine resulted in a polymer, provoking high antibody response in either strain. Genetic analysis of the response of F1 hyrids between high and low respond-

ers indicated that the immune response is under simple Mendelian
genetic control. These newly discovered genes, the immune response
(Ir) genes were extremely important in understanding the phenomena
of immunity and resistance to diseases. The same rules of genetic
control of the immune response apply also to native protein, but due
to their complexity, the phenomenon is noticed only under certain
limiting circumstances such as very low antigen doses, etc.

While the genetically controlled immune response is directed to
specific antigenic determinants, it has been observed already at an
early stage of the investigations that the chemical nature of the
carrier to which the determinant is attached is also of crucial importance. Furthermore, the whole phenomenon is linked to the major
histocompatibility locus of the immunized species. This could be the
basis for the linkage between various diseases, including auto-immune
diseases, and the main transplantation antigens in man, and also for
the varying response in different individuals to vaccination. Hence,
it might become an important factor in planning new vaccines in the
future.

SYNTHETIC ANTIVIRAL VACCINES

The feasibility of eliciting anti-protein immune response by
immunizing with a synthetic peptide conjugate, prompted the exploration of a similar approach for the induction of neutralizing antibodies against bacteria or viruses. In a model system of the bacteriophage MS-2, an immunologically active 20-amino acid residues synthetic peptide attached to a synthetic carrier did provoke antibodies
capable of efficiently inactivating the native bacteriophage. Furthermore, when the synthetic adjuvant MDP was attached to this conjugate it yielded a completely synthetic molecule that induced high
anti-phage neutralizing response even when injected in aqueous saline. Similar results were obtained for the diphtheria toxin, when
anti-toxic protective immunity was achieved by immunization with a
synthetic conjugate containing a 14 amino acid residue synthetic
fragment of the toxin.

A synthetic vaccine was also prepared against the microorganism
streptococcus pyogenes which is responsible for wide spread infections that cause complications such as rheumatic fever. A synthetic
peptide of 35 amino acid residues provoked in rabbits antibodies
that not only interact with the intact bacterium, but could confer
in mice passive immunity towards challenge infection.

The chemical synthetic approach has also proved effective for
some animal viruses such as hepatitis, foot and mouth disease and
influenza. In the case of hepatitis B, thirteen peptides have been
synthesized, with sequences covering most of the virus envelope
protein molecule, particularly the hydrophilic domains. Several of

these peptides induced in rabbits an immune response towards the native envelope protein of Dane particles of the hepatitis B virus. Another system tackled by this approach is foot and mouth disease. Synthetic peptides from two regions of one of the viral proteins produced high levels of serotype specific virus neutralizing antibodies in cattle, guinea pigs and rabbits. Moreover, a single inoculation of one of these peptides elicited sufficient neutralizing antibodies to protect guinea pigs against subsequent infection with the virus with approximately 10% efficiency of the intact virus particle. In the case of influenza, a fragment of the hemagglutinin molecule was synthesized, which comprises a common sequence for several strains of influenza subtype A. A conjugate of this peptide with tetanus toxoid induced in rabbits antibodies that reacted immunochemically with the peptide as well as with the intact virus of the relevant strains. The antibodies inhibited the hemagglutinin activity of this virus, and also interfered with its plaque formation in vitro. And foremost, immunization of mice with this conjugate resulted in partial protection against a challenge infection. It is thus apparent that synthetic materials can indeed lead to protective immunity against viruses, and hopefully against other disease causing agents, including bacteria and parasites.

SYNTHETIC ADJUVANTS

An important consideration in all vaccines is the adjuvant they contain in order to augment the immunogenicity of the primary agent. This point is even more crucial when synthetic vaccines are considered, since most of these substances are water soluble and tend to be less immunogenic than particulate materials. For experimental immunization in laboratory animals, the most commonly used adjuvant is Freund's complete adjuvant (FCA), which contains killed mycobacteria dispersed in a water-in-oil emulsion. It usually evokes high-level and long-lasting immunity. This adjuvant, however, is too problematic and is not adequate for use in humans since it induces local reactions, probably due to the very slow metabolic removal, if any, of the mineral oil and to the inflammation caused by the mycobacteria. Efforts have been made to replace this adjuvant by less damaging materials. A tremendous advancement has been achieved in this area, including the development of the synthetic adjuvant N-acetylmuramyl-L-alanyl-D-isoglutamine (or MDP for muramyl dipeptide) and its many analogs. Some of these materials were found to be adjuvant active when administered in an aqueous medium or even when given orally. Their strongest effect is when they are covalently attached to the immunizing antigen. It is therefore possible that the most effective vaccines of the future will be adequately designed completely synthetic materials-comprising a synthetic carrier, synthetic antigenic determinants of one or more disease causing agents, and a synthetic adjuvant.

It is thus evident that the field of synthetic antigens has progressed very far since its inception only two decades ago, and has developed from an isoteric subject dealing with hypothetically interesting materials into a most applied research topic that might lead to the vaccines of the future.

STRATEGIES FOR IMPROVING IMMUNOGENICITY:
THE DELIBERATE ASSOCIATION OF MHC (HLA) ANTIGENS
WITH OTHER MOLECULES

A.R. Sanderson

MRC Immunology Team, Nag's Head Yard Medical School
Guy's Hospital, London SE1 9RT
United Kingdom

Any effective, and general, way of augmenting the immunogenicity
of an antigen would constitute a major advance in immunology.
However, this worthwhile endeavour can be broken down into severel
different, albeit interrelated, components.

The presentation aspect is probably determined principally by
the physical form of the antigen, and by the route of administration.
The pioneering studies of Freund (1,2) showed that water-in-oil
emulsions act as particularly efficient adjuvants to an antigen present in the aqueous phase. If dried, heat-killed Mycobacterium tuberculosis organisms are incorporated into the oil phase of such
emulsions, the well-known Freund's Complete Adjuvant results, with
its attendant dramatic increase in potency over other techniques for
involving both cellular and humoral responses (3,4,5). Antigen precipitated, and thereby dispersed, with aluminium hydroxide floccules,
similarly enjoys an elevated response profile compared with presentation as a saline solution. The effectiveness of either method probably owes much to a slow release from the depot of antigen injected, together with the protection from denaturation or degradation
conferred by insolubility and a failure to disperse. The effect is,
therefore, to prolong the time that lower concentrations of material
are able to interact with the lymphoid system of the host. Essentially similar considerations apply to the route of administration.

The use of M. tuberculosis or other microorganisms exploit in
addition either the previous immunological history of the host, or
the central pharmacological and non-specific activation of cells of
the immune system by some microorganisms.

Somewhat different concepts began to be introduced when the es-

119

sential feature of co-operation was revealed in immune responses (6). T-cell help involves determinants on a polyepitopic antigen different from those against which the specific antibody is produced by B-cells or their progeny (7). In addition, it has been shown that co-operation at the cellular level is intimately linked to products of the Major Histocompatibility Complex (MHC) (8). Although the precise nature of the association between MHC molecules and any given antigen or epitope is not yet determined, certain features have emerged clearly. In some early stages of an immune response in mice, interaction of macrophages and B lymphocytes with helper T-cells appear to be most efficiently mediated by products of I-region loci (Class 2 molecules?) of the murine MHC, in consort with antigen. Somewhat differently, and at the other end of the immune response spectrum, when virus invoked cytolytic killer T-cells destroy their target, only infected cells sharing K or D locus products (Class 1 molecules) with the infected stimulating cell are killed (9). The conclusion is that the immunogenic epitopes of an antigen enjoy an intimate and specific relationship with MHC molecules throughout the immune response from recognition of foreignness to delivery of an immune mechanism. This relationship of so-called MHC restriction with antigens is not yet defined in precise structural terms. Nevertheless, a clear and strong association with some MHC Class I molecules have been established in some specific cases (15), although restriction implications have not been examined.

Earlier evidence indicated that any model for T-cell receptors and self recognition must account for the high frequency of immunologically competent cells showing specificity for allohistocompatibility molecules (10). Taking both MHC restriction within an animal, and the high frequency of allohistocompatibility reactivity between animals, into account, we hypothesised that if a foreign epitope could be deliberately associated with an MHC molecule, it would enjoy peculiar immune status.

Evidence in support was obtained from the immune response to human β2-microglobulin (hβ2M) in primates (11). β2M is the <u>essentially</u> invariant chain of Class I MHC molecules within all species so far examined. Although β2M is a carefully preserved molecule, evidence has been produced for dimorphism in mice and suggested in rats. Nevertheless hβ2M is likely to be very similar to primate β2M. Therefore, it was predicted that any immune response to hβ2M alone would probably be of low intensity in primates. This proved to be the case (Table 1). By contrast, and quite unexpectedly at the time, a much lower dose of hβ2M (by 100-fold), but presented in the form of a Class I MHC (HLA) molecule proved to be exceptionally immunogenic in the same species of primate (Table 1). It was suggested at the time that the association of hβ2M (in HLA molecules) with the Class I MHC chain conferred a unique immunogenicity on any epitopes present in hβ2M but absent in the primate concerned. It was the specific association with the human Class I alloantigen chain that con-

Table 1.   Immunogenicity of human β2-Microglobulin in Macaca irus
           monkeys

Injected protein in Incomplete Freunds Adjuvant (μg)	Number of Boosts	β2M form	Anti β2M titre by Farr assay
50-100	6	Free	93±13
0.5-1.0	3	Bound as HLA antigen	2406±1295

ferred the property of augmented immunogenicity. Although it may be
argued that recognition is more likely to be associated in the early
stages of the immune response with Class 2 or HLA-D molecules, we
share the views of Klein (12) that a biologically important function
is unlikely to be uniquely restricted to a single class of molecule,
although that class may be quantitatively more efficient than another
at the job. The monkey, then, recognises the HLA Class I chain essentially as if it were an "allo" MHC molecule, mounts an unusually
potent response with many cells responding to the "allo" stimulus,
and regards the associated hβ2M also as a potent stimulus. Further
exploitation of this principle may seem limited, but there is a
particular way in which foreign epitopes can be associated with
Class I alloantigens.

In MHC molecules the bond between the alloantigen chain and β2M
is non-covalent. Nevertheless, it is strong enough to resist 3M-salt
extraction although not sodium dodecyl sulphate or guanidinium
hydrochloride. It was demonstrated some time ago (13) that hβ2M
could become associated with the surface of mouse lymphocytes, and
it was subsequently shown that the association was particularly
with Class I H2 alloantigen molecules.

We have expanded on this (14) and shown that iodinated hβ2M can
serve as a sensitive and specific probe for the H2 alloantigen
chain (Table 2). Furthermore, the probe can be associated with the
H2 chain by incubating a partially purified surface glycoprotein
fraction with ^{125}I-β2M, or more simply by incubating intact, normal
or tumour cells (5-10x10^6) at about 2x10^7 per ml in 0.5ml medium
with 0.1 μg ^{125}I-labelled hβ2M at 160 μCi per μg for one hour at
37°C.

After brief washing with saline to remove unabsorbed ^{125}I-β2M,
cells are extracted with detergent to provide labelled H2 molecules

Table 2.   Incorporation of ^{125}I human β2M into mouse class I
           H-2 antigens

Antisera	Antigen recognized	AKR/J Intact lymphocytes (NP40 lysate)[†]	
		cpm	Percent total
Normal mouse serum		41	0.4
Anti-H-2.23	K^k	4056	42.1
Anti-H-2.32	D^k	1767	18.4
Anti-H-2.2	D^b	85	0.9
Anti-H-2.33	K^b	70	0.7
Anti-H-2.18	K^r	69	0.7
Anti-H-2.30	D^q	79	0.8
Normal rabbit serum		322	3.3
Rabbit anti-H-2	K,D	6741	70.1
Monoclonal antibodies		6237	62.8
Anti-H-2^k	K^k,D^k		
Anti-human β2m	BBM1 β2m(hu)	7209	74.9

[†] Precipitated using Protein A from S.aureus and appropriate
antiserum.

in solution which behave precisely as expected in several serological
assays testing for xenospecific β2M, xenospecific anti-H2 molecules,
or allo-specific H2 molecules. Control values range from 2.5-3.3% of
experimental results using anti-mouse globulin or protein A as the
precipitating system.

Success in this xenospecific system prompted us to examine other
probes of hβ2M for their ability to associate with HLA molecules.
This was achieved with considerable ease in solution using highly
purified HLA molecules. When the probe is radioactive as in the case
of ^{125}I or ^{3}H-dinitrophenol groups, association of altered hβ2M with
the HLA chain is easily detected by the change in size (11.6 Kilo-
daltons-45 Kilodaltons). Separation of unbound from bound labelled
hβ2M was achieved by gel filtration and counting of radioactivity
in fractions. In anticipation of attaching peptides or even proteins
to the hβ2M moiety of an HLA molecule, a heterobifunctional coupling
agent (m-maleimidobenzoyl N-hydroxysuccinimide ester) has also been
attached by acylation of an NH_2 group (presumably ε amino lysine)
in hβ2M.

Examination of the association and dissociation of labelled hβ2M with HLA molecules yielded some surprising findings. First, evidence was obtained that more than one derivatised hβ2M molecule could associate with the HLA chain. However, in all cases such complexes were not very stable in physiological saline and rechromatography yielded combinations where a stoichiometric ratio of 1 between HLA and hβ2M was obtained. Second, there appears to be a preferential association of the allospecific chain in HLA, or its analogue in other species, for altered hβ2M. Two examples of this are hβ2M which has been iodinated (^{125}I) and dinitrophenylated (^{3}H-DNP), which then exchanges particularly efficiently into xenospecific lymphocyte surfaces. Apart from mouse and rat we have also found the same for ^{125}I-hβ2M exchange into the surface of cow peripheral lymphocytes.

Of course, these results were obtained principally with radiolabelled hβ2M. However, it is important to appreciate that not all probes were present in trace amounts of nuclide. With ^{3}H-DNP-hβ2M the presence of an excess of unlabelled DNP-hβ2M allowed the preparation of isolatable HLA molecules unequivocally associated with DNP-hβ2M.

Preliminary results in primates (A.R. Sanderson unpublished) using HLA –hβ2M-DNP indicate (Table 3) that substantially augmented immunogenicity is provoked to the DNP moiety, which is present (on average) only once per HLA molecule and was inoculated only in Incomplete Freund's Adjuvant. Clearly these results require substantiation with other examples but the principle already appears promising and exciting.

Table 3. Augmented immunogenicity to the DNP moeity in primates

Antigen	Antibody Titre[†] in Primates		
	Prime	Boost 1	Boost 2
DNP-Ovalbumin	0	0	0
DNP (β2M)-HLA	100	1250	1650
DNP-β2M	0	325	250

[†] Tested on sheep erythrocytes sensitised with DNP in the form of dinitrophenylated (DNP) Fab of rabbit anti-sheep erythrocyte serum. Lysis was measured using rabbit complement. Titre given is the 50% end point using ^{51}Cr-labelled sheep erythrocytes. (A.R. Sanderson, unpublished).

REFERENCES

1. Freund, J. and McDermott, K., <u>Proc</u>. <u>Soc</u>. <u>Exp</u>. <u>Biol</u>., N.Y.
    49:548 (1942).
2. Freund, J., Thompson, K.J., Hough, H.B., Sommer, H.E. and
    Pisani, T.M., <u>J</u>. <u>Immunol</u>. 60:383 (1948).
3. White, R.G., Jenkins, G.C. and Wilkinson, P.C., <u>Int</u>. <u>Arch</u>.
    <u>Allergy</u> 22:156 (1963).
4. White, R.G., Coons, A.H. and Connolly, J.M., <u>J</u>. <u>Exp</u>. <u>Med</u>.
    102:83 (1955).
5. Nicol, T., McKelvie, P. and Druce, C.G., <u>Nature</u> 190:418 (1961).
6. Mitchison, N.A., <u>Eur</u>. <u>J</u>. <u>Immunol</u>. 1:18 (1971).
7. Rajewsky, K., Roelants, G.E. and Askonas, B.A., <u>Eur</u>. <u>J</u>. <u>Immunol</u>.
    2:592 (1972).
8. Julius, M.H., <u>Immunology</u> <u>Today</u> 3:295 (1982).
9. Zinkernagel, R.M. and Doherty, P.C., <u>Adv</u>. <u>Immunol</u>. 27:51 (1980).
10. Simonsen, M., <u>Cold</u> <u>Spring</u> <u>Harbor</u> <u>Symp</u>. <u>Quant</u>. <u>Biol</u>. 32:517
    (1967).
11. Sanderson, A.R., <u>Nature</u> 269:414 (1977).
12. Klein, J., Juretic, A., Baxevanis, C.N., Nagy, Z.A., <u>Nature</u>
    291:455 (1981).
13. Hester, R.B., Kubo, R.T. and Grey, H.M., <u>Scand</u>. <u>J</u>. <u>Immunol</u>.
    9:125 (1979).
14. Schmidt, W., Festenstein, H., Ward, P.J. and Sanderson, A.R.,
    <u>Immunogenetics</u> 13:483 (1981).
15. Signas, C., Katze, M.G., Persson, H. and Philipson, L., <u>Nature</u>
    (in press) (1982).

IMMUNOMODULATION IN TUMOR SYSTEMS

A. Matter[†]

Immunology Laboratories France
Schering Plough Corporation
69572 Dardilly, France

INTRODUCTION

This brief article is mainly concerned with the problems of
validity and reproducibility of animal tumor models when testing
defined pharmacological compounds. The questions that arise are:

Is there an immune response with cytostatic or cytotoxic potential against a tumor?

Is there a simple parameter with which to measure overall immune
anti-tumor activity?

Can this parameter be manipulated at will and reproducibly by
reference drugs?

And is the activity of a test drug against the tumor itself
clearly separable from its effect on the immune system?

In accordance with other authors, I think that at present the
syngeneic transplantable mouse tumor, injected intradermally (i.d.)
probably represents a useful model in various respects and may prove
to be valid in the future if the conclusions drawn from this type
of model prove to be borne out instance by clinical experimentation.
In fact, intradermal injection, in contrast to intraperitoneal
(i.p.) injection for instance, shows characteristics that strongly

---

[†] The work reported here was done while still at F. Hoffmann–La
Roche, Pharma–Research Division, Basel, Switzerland.

suggest an immune response during an early phase of tumor growth,
usually around day 7-15 after inoculation. This plateau leads to an
easily detectable stabilisation of tumor size, a most convenient
parameter for daily measurements in the intact host.

MATERIAL AND METHODS

Animals and Tumor Lines

    Source of inbred mice used and various transplantable murine
tumor cell lines have been described earlier (1-4).

Pharmacological Substances Used

    These comprise three classes and were all synthesized by the
chemical research department at Hoffmann-La Roche, Basel. (In brackets
{ } the number of the compound is shown).

a.   muramyl dipeptides

    5 different substances were produced:

    - N-acetyl-muramyl-L-alanyl-D-isoglutamine {1}
    - N-acetyl-muramyl-D-alanyl-L-isoglutamine {2}
    - N-acetyl-1.6-anhydro-muramyl-L-alanyl-D-isoglutamine {3}
    - N-acetyl-muramyl-L-alanyl-methyl-D-isoglutamine {4}
    - N-acetyl-muramyl-L-alanyl-D-glutamyl-L-tyrosine {5}

b.   alkyl-lysophospholipids

    - 1-octadecyl-glycero-3-phosphocholine {6}, Ro 14-0859
    - 1-octodecyl-2-methyl-glycero-3-phosphocholine {7}, Ro 14-5243

c.   vitamin A analogs (= retinoids)

    - retinoic acid {8}
    - ethyl all-trans-9-(4-methoxy-2,3,6-trimethyl-phenyl) 3,7-di-
      methyl-2,4,6,8-nonatetraenoate {9}, Ro 10-9359
    - all trans ethyl-9-(2,6-dichlor-4-methoxy-m-tolyl)-3,7-dime-
      thyl-2,4,6,8-nonatetraenoate {10}, Ro 12-7554

MODEL SYSTEMS

    The following systems have been used as described earlier
(1,3-5), to test compounds.

a. In vitro systems

    - Direct antiproliferative effect on tumor cells
    - Effect on mitogen-induced proliferation of lymphoid cells
    - Effect on the mixed lymphocyte culture
    - Effect on the generation and cytotoxic activity of the fol-
      lowing cells: NK cells, macrophages, ADCC- and cytotoxic T
      cells.
    - Effect on the memory of cytotoxic T cells.

b. In vivo systems

    Tumor models: number of cells injected are indicated in the
    figures. Routes of injection were intradermal, intraperitoneal,
    subcutaneous (neck and footpad). Parameters measured were the
    size of the tumor and/or ratio of dead versus surviving animals
    over time. Arbitrarily, a limit of 30 days was set after which,
    according to our experience, the ratio of tumor-bearing mice
    versus cured animals did not change anymore and animals were
    killed.

    Graft-versus-host and host-versus-graft reaction: this was in-
    duced in the footpad by injecting allogeneic cells into F1 or
    semiallogeneic cells into parent animals, respectively. Parameter
    measured was the weight of draining lymph node.

    Allogeneic (tumor) graft rejection: at the height of rejection,
    cytotoxic T lymphocytes were harvested from the peritoneal cavity
    and their number and relative activity measured in each animal
    using standard chromium release assays.

    Cell-mediated cytotoxicity: animals pretreated in vivo with test
    compounds were tested for NK, ADCC and macrophage-mediated cyto-
    toxicity against a panel of tumor cell targets.

    Adaptive transfer of cytotoxic T memory: highly irradiated ani-
    mals were inoculated with tumor cells and treated adoptively
    with unirradiated syngeneic immune cells from animals undergoing
    tumor rejection.

RESULTS AND DISCUSSION

    Figure 1 shows the development of tumor after intradermal injec-
tion in CBF1 mice. 10^6 syngeneic Meth-A sarcoma cells were injected
i.d. in a volume of 50 µl. Tumor size was measured three times
weekly.

    Several observations can be made: all animals develop tumor
initially at the same rate. After about 7 days growth slows markedly.

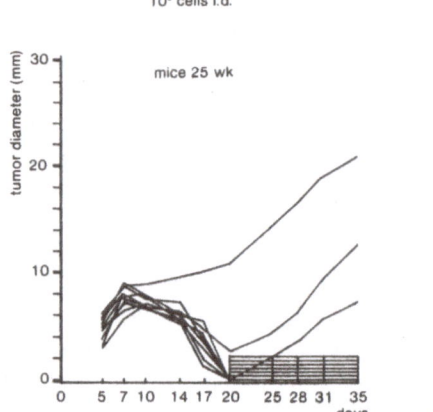

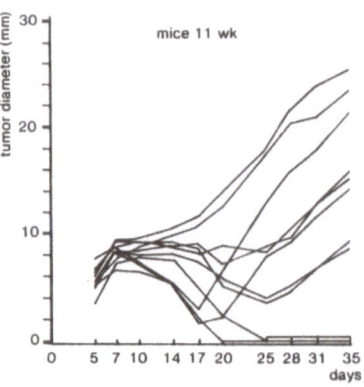

Fig. 1.   Measurement of tumor size in CBF1 mice after i.d. injection
of 10^6 syngeneic Meth-A sarcoma cells in a volume of 50 µl.
Tumor size was measured three times weekly.

Animals then divide into regressors and progressors. It is quite
remarkable to see that in some cases tumor can regress to undetec-
able levels and nevertheless can take off again and kill the animal.
Once tumor had disappeared for one week or longer, the animal could
be considered cured. In addition, this experiment shows the effect
of age: older animals seem less susceptible to tumor growth and show
a statistically significant higher proportion of regressors.

    Another point which merits attention is the choice of graphical
representation. Since the animal population behaves in a heterogeneous way (progressors vs regressors) mean values and standard de-
viations are meaningless. We have therefore chosen to show individual
growth curves on illustrations. Rank tests were used for statistical
analysis.

    Figure 2 shows three things: firstly, the instability of the
tumor line. Subline A and B are derived from the same Meth-A sarcoma
line propagated in vivo by Dr. Munder at the Freiburg Max-Planck
Institute. Subline A was kept in vivo during several months at
Hoffmann-La Roche in Basel in s.p.f. CBF1 mice. The difference in
"virulence" of the 2 sublines, which were tested in one batch of
mice from Basel is striking. Conversely, the subline B from Freiburg
grew faster in mice from the Freiburg mouse colony (data not shown).
Independently from the major histocompatibility type of a host we

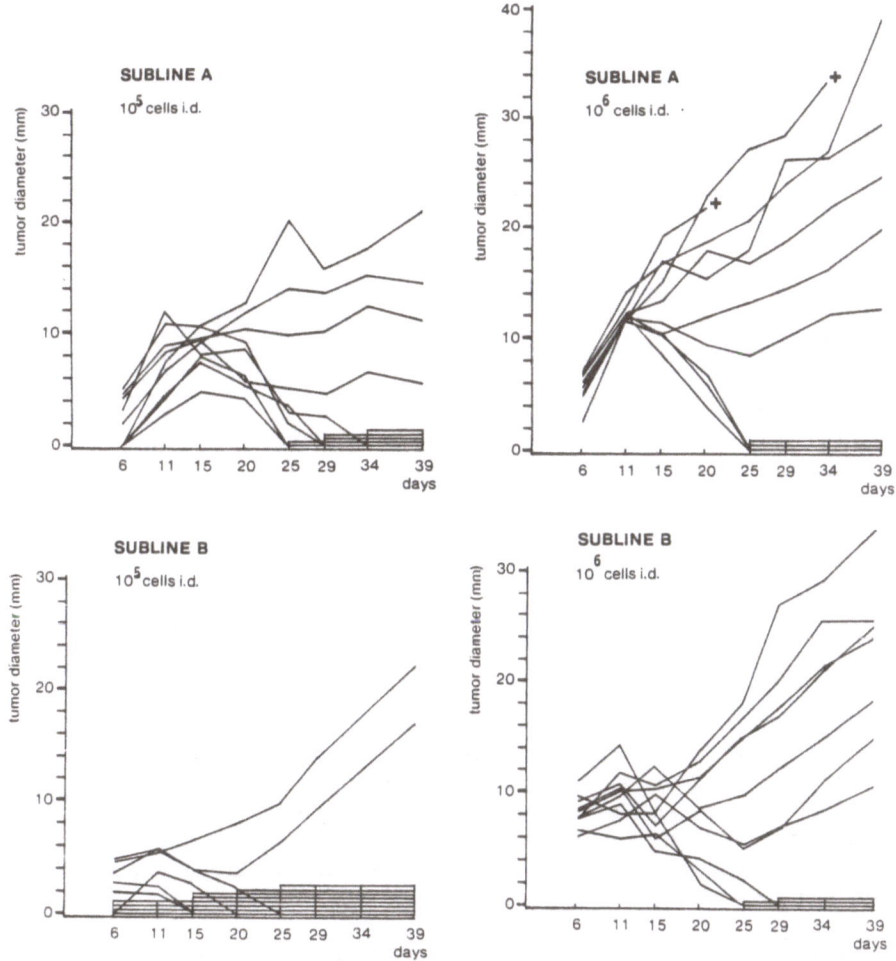

Fig. 2.   Measurement of tumor size in one batch of mice after i.d.
injection of subline A or subline B, both derived from
Meth-A sarcoma cells.

see an adaptation of a tumor to a particular host. The mechanism for
this is unknown. Secondly, initial growth and progression at late
stages are dependent on the number of inoculated tumor cells. This
is surprising since it could be argued that if tumor cell growth
proceeded as in vitro (doubling time approx. 14 hours) a 10-fold
difference in the size of inoculum would be erased within 2 days;
this is clearly not so and points to secondary mechanisms affecting
tumor growth. Thirdly it can be seen that in cases where tumor growth

Table 1. Effect of x-irradiation on a syngeneic tumor
          model[†]

Dose of x-irradiation	Progressors/ Regressors
nil	1/9
100 rad	5/5
200 rad	6/4

[†] 10^5 Meth-A sarcoma cells were injected intradermally
into (balb/c x C57 Bl/6) F_1 mice.

is very rapid the plateau phase is missing. Again, similarly as
above, host factors might be involved; it is probably not unreason-
able to suggest that an immune response is responsible for the plateau phase and this response is somehow overwhelmed by inocula that
exceed its capacity to react.

Table 1 further supports the idea of immune phenomena influencing
this tumor model; small doses of x-irradiation significantly decrease
the number of regressors. Undoubtedly the best argument is the immunity which can be achieved in this model: regressor animals are
protected during a period of about 23 months against the same tumor
even when injected i.p., a route which in the normal animal invariably leads to death (data not shown).

Similar data as the ones demonstrated in the Meth-A sarcoma in
CBF1 mice can be obtained with other tumors, always in the syngeneic
host: RBL-3, EL-4, P-815, YAC-1 and others.

It is this type of model that we attempted to influence pharma-
cologically. In order to gain insight into mechanisms we have first
examined the effects of a testcompound on the known cytotoxic effector cells with respect to their proliferative and differentiative
cycles as well as their cytotoxic activity itself. Secondly we have
tried to correlate this immunopharmacological profile with the anti-
tumor activity in vivo of a given test compound.

a. Muramyldipeptides (compounds {1-5})

With regard to adjuvant activity and all other activities mentioned below, only compound {1} was active (5). Proliferative T cell

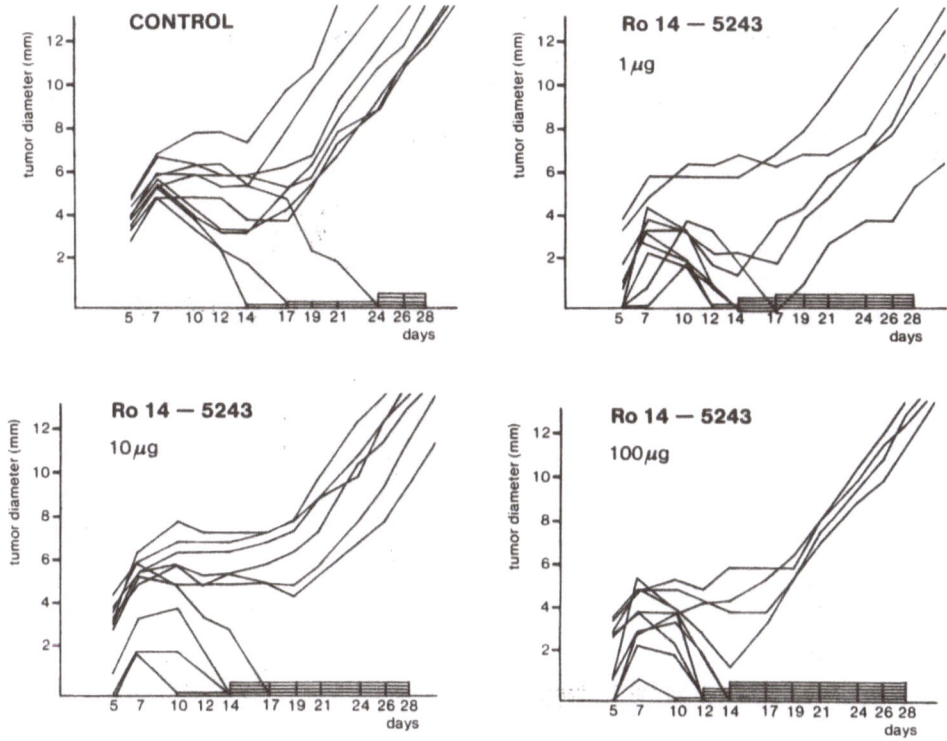

Fig. 3. Effect of different doses of Ro 14-5243 on tumor growth of Meth-A sarcoma cells in transplanted mice.

responses were enhanced, as well as the allogeneic cytotoxic T cell response in vivo. Activity of preformed cytotoxic T cells as well as cytotoxic T memory was unaffected. Macrophage-mediated and antibody-dependent cell cytotoxicity were both enhanced when cells were pre-treated in vivo. NK activity was decreased under these conditions. Despite this interesting profile it was impossible to define an anti-tumor activity of MDP (compound {1}). Eight separate experiments were performed involving four different syngeneic tumor models and i.p., i.v. and p.o. administration of dosages of MDP ranging between 10 μg and 10 mg/injection. Treatment was done on days 1, 1-4, or 1-7 after tumor inoculation. Each treatment group comprised 10 animals. Some slight effects were observed, these were sometimes enhancing, sometimes suppressing tumor growth, but not reproducibly so. In con-clusion it can be said that MDP alone is probably inactive in cur-rently used tumor models. MDP incorporated into liposomes seems to be able to generate macrophage cytotoxicity (6).

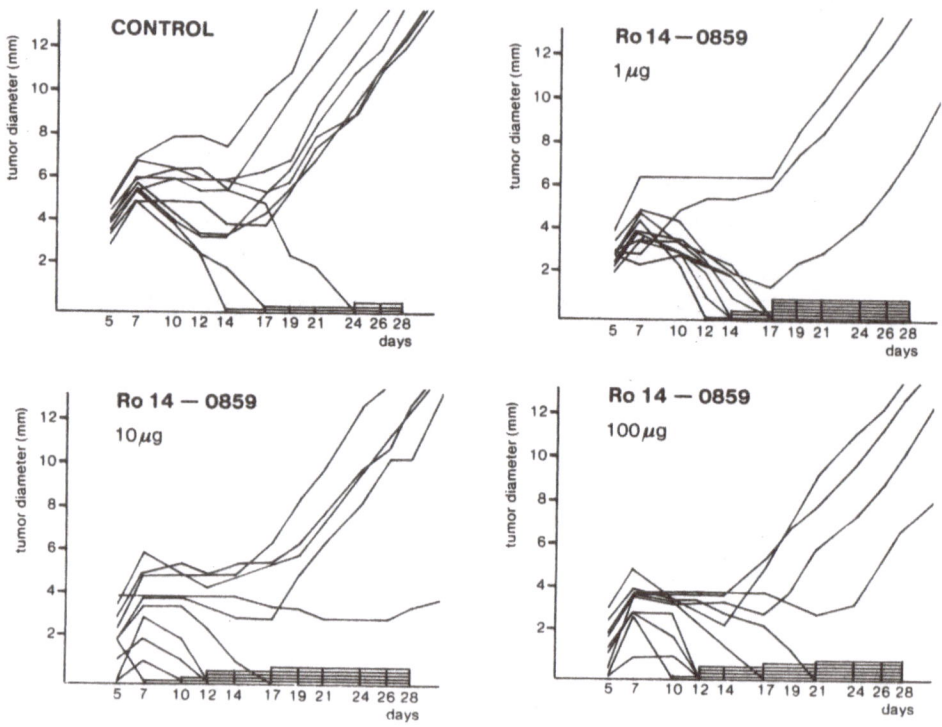

Fig. 4.   Effect to different doses of Ro 14-0859 on tumor growth of
          Meth-A sarcoma cells in transplanted mice.

b.   Alkyl-lysophospholipids

     These compounds have been invented by Dr. Munder and colleagues
(7) and show interesting activities in a variety of systems (8).
Beside their adjuvant activity they are able to increase in vivo
cytotoxic T cell activity and macrophage cytotoxicity. Interestingly,
and in contrast to MDP, these compounds do not act via enhanced proliferation; on the contrary, they exert in vitro direct antiprolifer-
ative effects on certain types of tumor cells.

     In vivo it is much more difficult to discern the anti-tumor po-
tential of lysophospholipids. There is certainly an effect; but it
is relatively weak and lacks dose dependence (Figures 3 and 4).
Other tumors such as B16, P-815, L1210 and RBL-3 are totally insen-
sitive to these substances and may even be enhanced. In the light
of these findings clinical experimentation with these compounds in
the tumor field must appear problematic.

Table 2. Treatment of syngeneic tumor with 2 retinoids[†]

Exp. no.	compound tested	dose mg/kg	Tumor-diameter in mm	% of control	% difference	significance at p value
	nil	---	12.40	100	---	
1	Ro 10-9359	3	10.75	87	-13	0.0005
	Ro 10-9359	30	8.17	66	-34	0.0005
	Ro 12-7554	3	7.10	57	-43	0.0005
	Ro 12-7554	30	8.67	70	-30	0.0025
	nil	---	11.40	100	---	
2	Ro 10-9359	3	10.85	95	-5	0.20
	Ro 10-9359	30	10.95	96	-4	0.20
	Ro 12-7554	3	11.40	100	0	---
	Ro 12-7554	30	10.35	91	-9	0.20
	nil	---	10.90	100	---	
3	Ro 10-9359	3	8.39	77	-23	0.0005
	Ro 10-9359	30	8.22	75	-25	0.0005
	Ro 12-7554	3	8.35	77	-23	0.0005
	Ro 12-7554	30	7.13	65	-35	0.0005
	nil	---	9.85	100	---	
4	Ro 10-9359	3	7.95	81	-19	0.0005
	Ro 10-9359	30	9.95	101	-1	0.45
	Ro 12-7554	3	11.20	114	-14	0.0025
	Ro 12-7554	30	8.45	86	-14	0.0025

[†] Measurements of tumor size 14 days after intradermal injection of 10^4 P-815 cells in DBA/2 mice. 10 animals/group. Treatment was done per os on days 4,6 and 8 after inoculation.

c. Retinoids

It is an old finding of Dresser et al. (9) that vitamin A has an
adjuvant effect on humoral immune responses. Felix et al. (10) and
Tannock et al. (11) described increased tumor resistance based on
immunological mechanisms due to vitamin A and, more recently, Dennert
et al. (12) and Lotan and Dennert (13) described increased T cell
cytotoxicity due to treatment with retinoids. Our own results confirm these results, though the effects observed were much less impressive than those obtained by above-mentioned investigators.

We have studied the effect of 2 retinoids in vivo in a syngeneic
tumor model (Table 2). The two retinoids chosen were active in a
variety of other systems (for review see Bollag and Matter, ref. 14).
Table 2 illustrates the typical pattern of results one obtains. 2
out 4 experiments show no effect, 2 others, strictly parallel experiments show a moderate effect, albeit with no dose-effect relationship. It is tempting in these circumstances to exclude some experiments on "technical" grounds and to select those that best fit the
bias of the investigator. At present it should be stressed that the
causes for this lack of reproducibility are unknown and most likely
are to be found in the inherent instability of host-tumor interaction. Neither tumor nor host are fixed entities; additionally, a
test compound is affecting several parameters of the immune system
simultaneously. This complexity is not understood at present. The
rationale for using defined pharmacological compounds lies in a
detailed analysis and comparison of in vitro and in vivo effects
in systems that are less complex.

In conjunction with chemical analogue series and pharmakokinetic
as well as biochemical data valuable conclusions can be drawn on the
contribution of a particular component to the overall anti-tumor
response. It is by this painstaking effort that we can hope to arrive
at an understanding of the constantly changing balance of forces in
tumor disease.

1. Matter, A., Transplantation 22:184 (1976).
2. Matter, A., Cell. Immunol. 37:107 (1978).
3. Matter, A., Immunology 36:179 (1979).
4. Hartmann, H.R., Matter, A., Cancer Res. 42:2412 (1982).
5. Matter, A., Cancer Immunol. Immunother 6:201 (1979).
6. Sone, S., Fidler, I.J., Cell Immunol. 57:42 (1981).
7. Munder, P.G., Weltzien, H.U., Modolell, M., in: "Immunopathology,
    VII International Symposium", P.G. Miescher, ed., Basel, p. 411
    (1977).
8. Runge, M.H., Andreesen, R., Pfleiderer, A., Munder, P.G.,
    J. Natl. Cancer Inst. 64:1301 (1980).
9. Dresser, D.W., Nature 217:527 (1968).
10. Felix, E.L., Loyd, B., Cohen, M.H., Science 189:886 (1975).

11. Tannock, I.F., Suit, H.O., Marshall, N., J. Natl. Cancer Inst.
    48:731 (1972).
12. Dennert, G., Crowley, C., Kouba, J., Lotan, R., J. Natl. Cancer
    Inst. 62:89 (1979).
13. Lotan, R., Dennert, G., Cancer Research 39:55 (1979).
14. Bollag, W., Matter, A., Annals NY Acad. Sciences 359:9 (1981).

IMMUNOMODULATION BY XENOBIOTICS: INTRODUCTORY

REMARKS TO IMMUNOTOXICOLOGY

Federico Spreafico, Annunciata Vecchi, Marina Sironi,
Walter Luini, Elena Pasqualetto, Miriam Romano, Anna
Merendino and Antonia Canegrati

Istituto di Richerche Farmacologiche "Mario Negri"
Via Eritrea, 62-20157 Milan, Italy

Immunotoxicology is the subspecialty concerned with the study
of the ill effects which result from the interaction of xenobiotics
with the immune system. Although these adverse effects can be the
consequence of an immune reaction to the foreign substance, we shall
here focus exclusively on the aspect of the damage inflicted by
xenobiotics on immunity.

In a paper of this length no attempts could be made to present
the current state of the art in this field in detail. We shall
therefore only discuss a number of selected general aspects while
referring to other publications for more extensive reviews including descriptions of the immune phenomenology associated with exposure to the various xenobiotics (1-4).

The use of immunological and host resistance assays has in
fact shown that animal exposure to a number of chemicals, drugs and
natural substances results in immune dysfunction modifying host resistance to challenges such as infectious agents and transplanted
tumors as well as producing alterations in the frequency of spontaneous neoplasms. Observations in selected populations of human
beings exhibiting immune derangements as a consequence of their
exposure to chemicals such as polyhalogenated biphenyls, have increased the awareness that the immune system can be a very sensitive target for the toxicity of foreign substances. This sensitivity essentially derives from the fact that many cell types of the
immune system continually undergo proliferation and differentiation,
and that physiological response depends on the harmonic interaction
of the various populations and subpopulations of immunocytes sus-

tained by a series of finely regulated networks. This complex organization provides thus a multiplicity of possible targets for cellular injury sustained not only by cell death but also by a variety
of possible functional derangements. It appears therefore reasonable
to suggest that an immunotoxicological evaluation should be included
in the routine toxicity assessment, and at the same time to emphasize that investigation of xenobiotics' effects on immune cells can
provide distinct advantages for dissection of mechanisms of cell
damage. In this the relative ease of obtaining various types of immunocytes and the possibility of assessing with sensitivity several
types of specialized cell activities are important factors.

A precise definition of immunotoxic substance has not yet been
produced. However, as discussed at more length elsewhere (4), a
series of aspects bearing on this problem have both practical and
conceptual importance and are thus worthy of mention. The first of
such aspects has to do with the fact that intrinsic in the concept
of immunotoxic substance is at least a degree of selectivity in the
effect exerted on the immune system vis-à-vis toxic effects exerted
on other systems. In other words, a xenobiotic can be regarded as
immunotoxic only if the immunological effects exerted are observed
at doses lower than those possessing general or other specific
pharmacotoxicological activity (e.g. hormonal) which may indirectly
influence immunoreactivity. A second aspect which should be emphasized is that, even though by far the majority of recognized immunotoxics are immunodepressants, xenobiotics causing enhanced expression of immunity, as for instance resulting from preferential or
exclusive damage to suppressor circuits, have also in principle to
be regarded as immunotoxics. It is further to be noted that,
although the immune derangement observed has to be of significant
magnitude and duration, it is not necessary that all types of immune
reactivity be concomitantly modified after exposure to a xenobiotic
for it to be rightly considered immunotoxic. As true also for im-
munotherapeutics (5), various foreign compounds have in fact been
shown to exhibit at least partial selectivity for the different populations and subpopulations of immune cells, and thus result in
change in one direction (e.g. depression) of given reactivities
coexisting with no changes, or even modifications in the opposite
direction (e.g. "enhancement"), in the expression of other types of
immune reactivity. For instance, administration to rodents of the
plant proteins MCI and PAP-S was associated with evident immuno-
depression sustained by functional inhibition of T cells, while B
cell function was untouched and macrophage function was markedly
enhanced (4). Treatment of mice with the tumor promoter phorbol
myristate acetate is associated with decreased T cell numbers and
thymus weight, reduced reactivity to T and B mitogens and antigens,
impaired NK cell function and reduced humoral responses and resistance to tumor challenges, concomitantly with increased macrophage
function and resistance to Listeria challenges (6).

Table 1. Immunotoxic Xenobiotics

Environmental Pollutants, e.g. polyhalogenated biphenyls
(PBBs, PCBs); TCDD, TCDF; styrene; phenol; vinyl chloride;
phtalates; dichloroethylene; hexachlorobenzene

Dusts, e.g. silica, carbon

Metal and salts, e.g. lead; cadmium; organic and inorganic compounds of mercury; Zn; Cr; Nio; CoSO4; chlorides of Ni, Mn, Cr, Cd;
organotins; arsenicals

Industrial solvents, e.g. propylenglycol

Pesticides, e.g. DDT; carbaryl; monuron; methyl parathion,
malathion, dichlorvos; dimethoate; hexachlorobutadiene;
orthophenylphenol

Carcinogens and promoters, e.g. polycyclic aromatic hydrocarbons;
phorbol esters; teleocidin

Plant and fungal products, e.g. aflatoxins; abrin; ricin; gelonin,
ochratoxins; PHA

Food additives, e.g. pyrogallol; vanillin, tartrazine carrageenan;
gallic a., butylhydroxytoluene

Drugs, e.g. anesthetic gases; steroid contraceptives;
diethylstillbestrol; phenobarbital; antiepileptics

Addictive substances, e.g. heroin; cannabinols; ethanol

Immune effects induced can therefore be complex, ranging from
coherent modifications in all expressions of the immune orchestra
to more selective damages. For instance, exposure of rodents to the
benz-a-pyrene results in severe depression of humoral immunity
whereas cell-mediated immunity is relatively spared (6). At
variance, exposure to two other carcinogens, diethylstilbestrol
and 3,4,7,8-tetrachlorodibenzodioxin (TCDD) caused depression in
both cellular and humoral reactivities (4,6), and treatment with
steroid contraceptive agents caused a selective impairment of T
cell function (4).

Immunotoxics have thus to be considered as a composite category of substances with marked qualitative and quantitative heterogeneity in their individual profiles. Although human data exist for
only a few substances (e.g. TCDD, polychlorimated biphenyls), a

Table 2. Minimal Panel of Assays for Screening Immunotoxic
          Xenobiotics in Rodents

Immunopathotoxicology	Hematology profile; lymphoid organ weights (spleen, thymus, lymph node)
Host resistance	Susceptibility to transplantable syngeneic tumor
Delayed cutaneous hypersensitivity	T-cell dependent antigen
Lymphocyte function	Blastogenesis to mitogens (PHA or Con A, LPS) and allogeneic lymphocytes (MLC)
Humoral Immunity	Immunoglobulin (IgM, IgG, IgA) levels, antibody plaque response to sheep erythrocytes

relatively high number of substances has been found to possess
definite immunotoxicological activity in experimental animals, as
exemplified in Table 1, which should by no means be contrued as an
exhaustive listing. It is apparent that this list encompasses compounds which are largely distributed in human micro or macroenvi-
ronment, a fact which should incite greater interest in the possible role of such substances in the pathogenesis of human or animal
disease. Table 1 also indicates that an immunological activity is
possessed by substances of widely different chemical structure and
origin. In this connection, it should be emphasized that chemicals
structurally closely related may nevertheless markedly vary in
their quantitative and/or qualitative interaction with immunity.
For instance, substantial differences in immunodepressive potency
was observed among steroid contraceptive agents as well as between
the polyhalogenated hydrocarbons TCDD and TCDF.

     With regard to qualitative differentials among chemical ana-
logues, evidence has been obtained with various immunodepressive
agents supporting the concept that not only immunocytes of different lineages can substantially vary in their in vivo or in vitro
sensitivity to damage by cytotoxic agents, but also that important
differences in this sensitivity may exist among subsets of immune
cells of the same lineage present in a given lymphoid organ (5).

     The selection of the minimal experimental systems for the ini-
tial recognition of the possible immunotoxicity of xenobiotics
(e.g. screening of a novel industrial product) is still one of the

major open problems of Immunotoxicology. Essentially, this stems
from the still very limited experience on the sensitivity, specificity, reproducibility and, especially, predictiveness for man of
the various animal tests so far employed (4). The complexity of the
immune apparatus, the multitude of parameters which can be evaluated
and our only imperfect knowledge of the significance of at least
certain parameters, suggest a preference for in vivo testing which
can be expected to be more "complete" and representative, rather
than the exclusive use of in vitro approaches, which although more
economical, suffer from a number of important shortcomings. This
general philosophy is that followed in the testing approach to immunotoxicity screening summarized in tables 2 and 3 (6), which
although shown generally predictive for a number of model compounds,
should still be considered essentially as a working proposal, currently under evaluation under the sponsorship of the Nat. Inst.
Environm. Health Sciences, NIH, USA. A detailed discussion of the
merits and limits of each of these tests is beyond the scope of
this article. It may suffice therefore to emphasize that a great
deal of work has still to be conducted before scientifically sound
guidelines identifying the minimal tests to be performed for con-
ducting an immunotoxicological screening with reasonable expecta-
tions of predictiveness within acceptable cost-time frameworks, can
be proposed.

In connection with this general problem, a number of points
have to be considered in the assessment of the immunological activity of xenobiotics. Among these factors is the possibility that
given immune reactivities may exhibit different sensitivity to modulation not only in different species but also in different
strains within a species. For instance, the humoral depression induced by TCDD in the mouse is markedly strain-dependent, exhibiting
a suggestive correlation with the number and/or affinity of specific membrane binding sites for this chemical (7). The bases for
these interspecies differences are in most cases unknown, but their
possible existence implies that more than one animal species should
be investigated in the objective of basing on firmer ground possible
extrapolations to man. For such extrapolations, comparisons should
be made on the basis of the levels of the xenobiotics in the body
rather than simply on the dose administered. For instance, saccharin
impaired T cell function in rodents but only at concentrations by
far in excess of those obtainable in man in realistic conditions of
exposure (8). If therefore realistic exposures as regards doses and
routes should be employed in animal testing of foreign compounds
aimed at determining the actual or potential immunotoxicity of
xenobiotics, the possibility should further be mentioned that human
and animal cells may differ intrinsically in their sensitivity to
foreign substances. Human lymphoid cells in vitro were unaffected
by levels of Saccharin definitely reducing rodent cells' functional
capacities. In this regard, the possibility of assessing in vitro
the function of human circulating immune cells of several types is

Table 3. More Comprehensive Immunotoxicology Screening Panel under
          Evaluation at N.I.E.H.S., NIH

Pathotoxicology	: Hematology profile (Hb, RBC, WBC, differential); clinical chemistry (CPK, α-HBDH, SGPT, creatinine, acid and alk. phosphatase, LDH, cholinesterase) serum proteins (alb., globulin, A/G, total proteins), weights (body, spleen, thymus, liver, kidney), histology (thymus, spleen, adrenal, heart, kidney, lung, liver)
Host Resistance	: Syngeneic tumor cell challenge, Lysteria monocytogenes challenge, endotoxin hypersensitivity, expulsion of Trichinella spiralis
Delayed hypersensitivity	: T-cell dependent antigen with radiometric assay
Lymphocyte proliferation	: Mitogens (PHA, Con A, LPS,) Unidirectional mixed lymphocyte culture
Humoral immunity	: Immunoglobulin (IgM, IgG, IgA) levels, antibody plaque response to T-dependent (SRBC) and independent (LPS) antigens
Macrophage function	: Resident peritoneal cell nos. and nonspecific esterase staining, phagocytosis, lysosomal enzymes (LAP, acid phosphatase, S' nucleotidase), cytostasis of tumor target cells, RES clearance (^{125}I-triolein)
Bone marrow colony-forming units	: CFU-S multipotent stem cell nos, CFU-GM (granulocyte-macrophage) progenitor cells nos., cellularity; ^{59}Fe incorporation in bone marrow and spleen

---

a distinct advantage of immunotoxicology vis-à-vis other toxicology
investigations. However, it should also be noted that immunocytes
of a given lineage but present in different lymphoid and non-lymphoid
organs may exhibit different sensitivities to modulation by exogenous compounds.

In a series of recent experimental studies (9), it has in fact
been shown that a number of immunodepressants variably affect the
functional capacity of various types of immunocytes (e.g. macrophages, NK and T cells) present in the circulation, in a standard
lymphoid district as the spleen, and in peripheral organs such as

the lung and the gut. Depending on the compound investigated, examples of both higher and lower sensitivity to damage in immune cells
of a given type taken from these peripheral organs viz. their coun-
terparts in spleen and/or blood, were seen.

As it is also true for the differential sensitivity to a given
substance observable among immunocytes of different populations and
subpopulations, the exact mechanistic bases for this inter-organ
differential observable with some but not all cytotoxic agents, are
in most cases still unclear. Presumably complex interplays among
factors still largely unexplored, and ranging from differences in
tissue levels of the xenobiotic and/or its biotransformation products, in the turnover rates of the target and/or respective regulatory immunocytes, to differences in intrinsic sensitivity of the
cells, are operative. Nevertheless, the possibility that measurement
of immune functions in cells taken from lymphoid organs or blood may
not be representative of what occurs in peripheral districts which
are the sites of the first encounter between the xenobiotic and the
host, highlights the importance of using realistic routes of exposure and of attempting to evaluate "peripheral" parameters of immunity in addition to systemic parameters in order to obtain more
detailed and representative pictures of the immunological activity
of exogenous substances.

The immunological effect of xenobiotics tends to wane with
time, the duration of the modification depending generally on the
dose administrated, the type of reactivity examined and host age at
the time of initial exposure. For instance, exposure of mice to
urethane results in early impairment of NK activity, responsiveness
to mitogens and splenocyte depletion, whereas at later times a
strong reduction in NK activity can be seen concomitantly with
normal lymphoid cellularity and responsiveness to polyclonal activators (3).

In adult mice given TCDD, macrophage numbers were decreased
only several days after thymus and spleen involution and decrease
in cellular and humoral immunity (8). Much lower doses of TCDD were
immunodepressive when given in the perinatal period than to young
adult mice, the former type of treatment resulting additionally in
reduction in the functional capacity of cells (e.g. NK) involved in
natural resistance, whereas no functional impairments in these
cells were seen with adult treatments although the total capacity
to express this and other types of cellular immunity was reduced
due to lymphoid depletion (8).

The use of very young animals, or of in utero treatments thus
exposing the developing immune system to the xenobiotic, can be an
important experimental variable not only for increasing the sensitivity of the testing conditions but also for obtaining a better
assessment of the immunotoxic potential of xenobiotics. A similar

type of reasoning would in general also be expected to apply also
to aged animals with an involuted immune system. The possibility
that moderate, per se pathologically subthreshold derangements induced by a xenobiotic may synergize with other immunomodifying influences (e.g. malnutrition, infectious agents) thus resulting in
overt pathology, should therefore not be overlooked. Relevant to
this point is the fact that with many chemicals repeated exposures
result in significant decreases in the threshold immunotoxic dose
compared to acute treatments, and with at least a number of compounds with long persistence in the body (e.g. TCDD) immune effects
can be very long-lasting even after single exposures to minute
amounts (micrograms) of a chemical.

In conclusion, a large number of substances of different origin,
nature and structure has already been identified as immunotoxic in
experimental conditions. As interest in this type of toxicity is
relatively new, it can reasonably be assumed that those described
constitute only a minority of existing xenobiotics possessing immune
activity.

The susceptibility of the immune system to a wide variety of
foreign substances to which man can be acutely or chronically exposed in real life under a variety of circumstances, together with
consideration of the pivotal role of an intact immunity in health
maintenance, justify more active interest in this type of studies.

As might have been expected in view of the complexity of the
system which offers a multiplicity of levels at which damage can be
exerted through a variety of mechanisms, immunotoxic substances so
far characterized have proven markedly heterogeneous in their immunological profiles, a point which reflects the fact that the various populations and subpopulations of immune cells can markedly
differ in their susceptibility to injury by exogenous compounds.
Immune effects induced can therefore be complex. Since a number of
factors can critically influence the immune activity of xenobiotics,
assessment of immunotoxicity is still a complex exercise in which
a number of both practical and conceptual problems are still unre-
solved, and requires integration between immunological and toxicological expertise. If greater attention should be paid to the possibility that immunomodulation by substances in human environment
may have a role in disease causation, damage to the immune system
can be a very sensitive indicator of toxicity, revealing noxious
activities with greater sensitivity than seen with currently available toxicological investigations of other systems.

Lastly, in view of the varied and complex nature of the activities sustained by lymphoid cells, immunocytes can be important
models for the study of toxic mechanisms of foreign substances,
whereas chemical agents can be useful probes for the dissection and
better definition of the complexities of the immune system.

REFERENCES

1. Vos, J.G., CBC Crit. Rev. Toxicol. 5:67–101 (1977).
2. Faith, R.E., Luster, M.I. and Vos, J.G., Rev. Biochem. Toxicol.
    2:175–212 (1980).
3. Dean, J.H., Luster, M.I. and Boorman, G.A., in:
    "Immunopharmacology", Sirois, P. and Rola-Pleszcynski, M.
    (eds.), Elsevier, Amsterdam, pp. 349–397 (1982).
4. Spreafico, F. and Vecchi, A., in: "Advances on Immunomodulators",
    Ambrogi, F. and Fudenberg, H.H. (eds.), Plenum Press, New York,
    (1983) (in press).
5. Spreafico, F., Tagliabue, A. and Vecchi, A., in:
    "Immunopharmacology", Sirois, P. and Rola-Pleszcynski, M. (eds.),
    Elsevier, Amsterdam, pp. 315–348 (1982).
6. Dean, J.H., Luster, M.I., Boorman, G.A. and Lauer, L.D.,
    Pharmacol. Rev. 34:137–148 (1982).
7. Spreafico, F., Vecchi, A., Sironi, M. and Filippeschi, S., in:
    "Proceedings International Symposium Immunotoxicology",
    Academic Press, New York (1983) (in press).
8. Spreafico, F., Vecchi, A., Mantovani, A., Tagliabue, A.,
    Sironi, M., Luini, W. and Garattini, S., in: "Advances in
    Immunopharmacology", Hadden, J., Chedid, L., Mullen, P. and
    Spreafico, F. (eds.), Pergamon Press, Oxford, pp. 295–310 (1981).
9. Spreafico, F., Alberti, S., Allegrucci, M., Canegrati, A.,
    Colotta, F., Luini, W., Pasqualetto, E., Romano, M., Sironi, M.,
    and Vecchi, A., in: "Advances in Immunopharmacology II",
    Hadden, J.W., Chedid, L. and Spreafico, F. (eds.) Pergamon
    Press, Oxford (1983) (in press).

ANTIBODY PRODUCING HUMAN-HUMAN HYBRIDOMAS

L. Olsson

Medical Department A
State University Hospital
Copenhagen, Denmark

INTRODUCTION

Monoclonal hybridoma antibody technology has already proven to
be highly useful in a variety of biological areas (1-3). Only a few
papers have reported on production of human monoclonal hybridoma
antibodies as produced by human-human hybridomas (4-7) and none of
these reports have dealt with the technical details of the human-
human hybridoma system. We here report on technical difficulties and
improvements of the human-human hybridoma system.

MATERIALS AND METHODS

The majority of the human-human fusions was carried out by
using a HAT-sensitive, EBV-negative human B-lymphoma line (RH-L4)
that produces, but does not secrete, low amounts of γ-heavy chain
and k-light chain; some experiments were done with a mycoplasma-
cleaned variant of the SKO-007 line. The human cell lines were maintained in RPMI-1640 medium with 15% fetal calf serum. All the human
fusions were done with human lymphoid cells from peripheral blood
and were carried out in 37% w/v polyethylene glucol (PEG), MW 1000
(Baker, U.S.A.) at room temperature. The cells were seeded at a
concentration of 2 x 10^5 cells/well in 96-well microtiter plates
(Nunc, Denmark) in HT-medium with 15% FCS and hybrid selection in
HAT-medium was started 24-48 hours after fusion. The importance of
optimal feeder cell sources for human hybridoma growth has been
described in detail elsewhere. Lymphoid cells were in some experiments mitogen-stimulated with pokeweed mitogen (PWM). Antibody
analyses were done by ELISA for Ig-production, cell-binding ELISA
for cell surface antigens, and FACS analysis also for cell-surface

147

antigens. Monoclonality of an antibody was assessed by 2D-analysis
and the isotype of the antibody determined by class specific antibodies in an ELISA.

RESULTS

100 human-human fusion experiments were done with the RH-L4
line 53. The frequency of hybrids varied from 7% to 70% in the
various experimental groups and so did the number of wells with
hybrids (4%-56%). The amount of fusions resulting in hybrids was
slightly higher with the RH-L4 line (39%) as compared to the SKO-007
line (19%), and the amount of wells with IgG/IgM production was significantly higher with RH-L4 fusions as compared to SKO-007 (51%
versus 35%; $p < 0.01$ with X^2-test). Among the 100 fusions, only 21
resulted in antibody producing hybrids and in these 21 fusions the
average amount of wells with Ig-producing hybrids were 11%. Only
fifteen wells contained antibody-producing hybrids with predefined
specificity out of 72 fusions (about 18 000 wells).

The amount of specific hybrids, as well as hybrids with specific Ig-production was thus very low as compared to conventional
mouse-mouse fusions with optimally antigen-primed spleen cells.
However, the relevant comparison between the two systems is to com-
pare the hybridoma yield, when mouse PBLs are fused with X63
Ag/8.6.5.3 and human PBLs fused with RH-L4 or SKO-007 cells. It was
found that very low yield of hybrids in the groups using mouse
PBLs. The 100 fusions resulted in 21 wells with hybrids producing
antibody against antigens with known specificity. Only 3 of these
21 cultures were successfully cloned and re-expanded. Human PBLs
are normally not in active cell cycle, and fusions of such cells
with a human myeloma/lymphoma cell line may therefore not result in
functional mononuclear hybridoma cells. PBLs were stimulated with
pokeweed mitogen (PWM) prior to fusion. The PWM-stimulation is done
in HAT-medium to adapt the lymphocytes to the DNA-synthesis rescue
pathway that the hybrids use to overcome the HAT-blockage. Forty
fusions of PWM-PBLs with RH-L4 resulted in 14 with hybrid growth,
which is significantly higher as compared with fusions of PBLs with
RH-L4 cells.

DISCUSSION

The rodent hybridoma system is highly dependent on optimal
antigen-primed B-lymphocytes (8). This can easily be obtained in
laboratory animals, whereas similar in vivo primed human B-lymphocytes are practically impossible to obtain in human beings. Out of
72 fusions and more than 18 000 wells only 3 cloned hybrid cultures
of interest were obtained. Obviously, this is dramatically lower
than the results obtained with mouse-mouse fusions using antigen-

primed spleen cells. However, our results also show that the correct comparison between the murine and human system (mouse PBLs fused with a mouse myeloma line versus human PBLs fused with human cells) give similar poor yield of hybrids in the mouse-mouse hybridoma system.

Mitogen stimulation of PBLs in HAT-medium as well as optimal feeder cell conditions greatly improved the hybridoma yield, although it remained significantly lower as compared to the traditional mouse system. We think that this difference is mainly due to suboptimal source of antigen-primed cells and to some extent to a suboptimal malignant fusion partner. It seems therefore of crucial importance for the human-human hybridoma system that optimal in vitro antigen-priming systems are developed.

REFERENCES

1. Kennett, R.H., McKearn, T.J., Bechtol, K.B. (eds.), Plenum Press, New York, p.1 (1980).
2. Hammerling, G.J., Hammerling, U., Kearney, J.F. (eds.), "Monoclonal antibodies and T-cell hybridomas", Elsevier, Amsterdam, p.1 (1981).
3. McMichael, A. and Fabre, J. (eds.), Academic Press, New York, p.1 (1982).
4. Olsson, L. and Kaplan, H.S., Proc. Natl. Acad. Sci. (USA), 77:5429 (1980).
5. Croce, C.A., Linnenbach, A., Hall, W., Steplewski, Z., Korpowski, H., Nature 288:488 (1980).
6. Sikora, K., Anderson, T., Phillips, J., Watson, J.V., Lancet 1:2 (1982).
7. Shoenfeld, Y., Hsu-Lin, S.C., Gabriels, J.E., Silberstein, L.E., Furie, B.C., Furie, B., Stoller, B.D., Schwartz, R.S., J. Clin. Invest. 70:205 (1982).
8. Oi, V.T., Jones, P.P., Goding, J.W., Herzenberg, L.A., Curr. Top. Microbiol. Immunol. 81:115 (1978).

LYMPHOCYTE DYSFUNCTIONS ASSOCIATED

WITH ENZYME DEFECTS

B.J.M. Zegers, L.J.M. Spaapen, W. Kuis, J.J. Roord,
G.T. Rijkers and J.W. Stoop

University Children's Hospital, Utrecht
The Netherlands

INTRODUCTION

Nowadays three heritable molecular defects have been recognized as the primary cause of the associated immune deficiency syndrome. Adenosine deaminase (ADA) deficiency usually is associated with Severe Combined Immunodeficiency (SCID), purine nucleoside phosphorylase (PNP) deficiency is associated with cellular immune deficiency and absence of transcobalamine II (TC II) is associated with agammaglobulinemia (as well as with defects in the cells of the erythropoietic and myelopoietic cell lineage) (1). These causal associations imply the involvement of purine (and pyrimidine) metabolism and of cobalamine in the development and function of the lymphoid system (2). A low activity of another enzyme of the purine metabolic pathway, i.e. ecto-5'-nucleotidase (ecto-5'-NT) has been found in the lymphocytes of patients with hypogammaglobulinemia (3). Meanwhile lymphocytic ecto-5'-NT has been shown to be a marker of the maturation stage of the lymphocytes and low lymphocyte ecto-5'-NT activity in hypogammaglobulinemia may reflect a maturation arrest of the lymphocytes in these patients (2,3). More recently an as yet unexplained association of lymphocytic ecto-5'-NT deficiency with the syndrome of Omenn and concurrent combined immune deficiency has been reported (4).

In addition to the deficiencies of ADA, PNP and TC II a number of other metabolic or biochemical abnormalities seem to be associated with disturbances of the development and function of the lymphoid system. For example the relation of zinc deficiency to immunological function has been clearly established (5). Furthermore, patients with abnormalities of branched chain aminoacid metabolism

151

Table 1. Clinical Features of Three Dutch PNP-Deficient Sisters

	H., $2\frac{1}{2}$ yrs[†]	R., $1\frac{1}{2}$ yrs[†]	Re, alive born in 1975
Recurrent infections of respiratory tract, skin	+	+	+
Other infections	progressive vaccinia		severe chickenpox protracted HBV-infection
Neurologic abnormalities	spastic tetraparesis	spastic tetraparesis	spastic tetraparesis cerebellar ataxia extra-pyrimidal syndrome
Megaloblastic bone marrow	+	?	+
Neutropenia	+	+	+
Treatment	fetal thymus transplantation		long-term enzyme replacement, deoxycytidine
Cause of death	lymphosarcoma	Graft-versus-host-disease	

due to lack of biotin-dependent carboxylases have been shown to present defects in T cell and B cell immunity (6,7).

This contribution deals with ADA-and PNP-deficiency with emphasis on the role of purine metabolism in T and B cell development and function.

CLINICAL AND IMMUNOLOGICAL CHARACTERISTICS OF ADA- AND PNP-DEFICIENCY

ADA-deficiency is present in approximately 30 to 50% of patients with the autosomal recessive form of SCID. 80 to 90% of ADA⁻-SCID-patients show the symptoms of classical SCID in the first six months of life; i.e. severe and recurrent infections with bacteria, fungi and viruses as well as failure to grow (and often chronic diarrhea). ADA⁻-SCID patients may have neurologic abnormalities (e.g. nystagmus and spasticity) as well as bony abnormalities. Clinical variability does occur with respect to the onset of the disease as well as to the associated findings of bony and neurological abnormalities. Furthermore, variability in the immunological features of ADA⁻-patients is recognized: e.g. some patients have B-lymphocytes which may function in vivo as well as in vitro. This indicates that T cell function is more severely impaired than B cell function. In many patients with ADA⁻-SCID the immunological defects become more severe with age, e.g. B cells and antibody production may disappear throughout the first year of life. This immunologic involution has been attributed to a gradually increasing damage of the lymphoid system (2,8).

Clinically, PNP-deficiency may manifest itself later in life than ADA-deficiency. The disease is inherited in an autosomal recessive way. Infections may appear from the second half of the first year and they are predominantly of viral nature. PNP-deficiency is associated with severely impaired proliferation-dependent T-lymphocyte functions, whereas T helper function and B-lymphocyte function as expressed in the synthesis of specific antibodies are, at least in part, intact in these patients. No bony abnormalities have been described. Similarly as mentioned for ADA-deficiency, the T cell dysfunction becomes more severely impaired with age (9). Table 1 illustrates the general clinical features: the findings in three PNP-deficient Dutch patients are given (10, 11, 12). A gradually decreasing T cell function could be documented in the third child (11). Serum immunoglobulin levels developed normally and specific antibodies against a number of viruses were detectable.

More than 30 families are known from literature with ADA-deficiency and concurrent SCID (or CID). At present 13 patients with PNP-deficiency (eight families including those discovered in England and Spain recently) have been described (9, 13, 14).

AETIOPATHOGENETIC MECHANISMS

ADA and PNP are involved in the catabolism of purine nucleotides. ADA converts adenosine into inosine. PNP converts inosine into hypoxanthine and guanosine into guanine. The enzymes both convert also the deoxy-compounds. The metabolic abnormalities in ADA- and PNP-deficiency are indicated in Table 2. ADA-deficient patients have markedly elevated adenosine (Ado) and deoxyadenosine (dAdo), the metabolites before the metabolic block, in their serum and urine. They accumulate deoxyadenosine triphosphate (dATP) in erythrocytes and more importantly in the lymphocytes (1,15). In addition the lymphocytes show increased concentrations of cyclic-AMP. PNP-deficient patients excrete large quantities of inosine,

Table 2. Metabolic Features of ADA and PNP-Deficiency

	ADA$^-$	PNP$^-$
plasma, urine	adenosine ↑	inosine ↑, deoxyinosine ↑
	deoxyadenosine ↑	guanosine ↑, deoxyguanosine ↑
erythrocytes	deoxy ATP ↑	deoxy GTP ↑
	SAH[+] ↓	SAH ↓
lymphocytes	deoxy ATP ↑	deoxy GTP ↑
	cyclic AMP ↑	

[+] SAH = S-Adenosylhomocysteine hydrolase (12,20)

deoxyinosine, guanosine (Guo) and deoxyguanosine (dGuo) and have elevated levels of these metabolites in the serum. In addition, they accumulate deoxyguanosine triphosphate (dGTP) in the erythrocytes (15) and the lymphocytes (16). Figure 1 shows the specific effects of PNP-deficiency: Guo and dGuo cannot be converted into guanine, they increase in the serum and are found in massive quantities in the urine. dGuo is phosphorylated into dGMP by deoxycytidine kinase which is predominantly -although not exclusively- present in the cells of the lymphoid system and in particular in thymocytes (17). The final product dGTP inhibits the reduction of cytidine diphosphate into deoxycytidine diphosphate (dCDP) by the enzyme ribonucleotide reductase. As a result dCTP is depleted in the lymphocytes and DNA-synthesis is hampered by lack of an essential DNA-precursor. As far as ADA-deficiency is concerned, recent findings on resting cells disclosed that the effect of lymphocytic dATP formation in this condition rather affects ATP levels than interference with ribonucleotide reductase (18,19). Furthermore, two additional mechanisms have been proposed for ADA-deficiency: cylic AMP mediated modulation of immune function, and Ado and dAdo mediated increase in S-adenosyl homocystein (20), an inhibitor of methylation reactions which are required for a number of cellular functions such as chemotaxis, cytotoxicity and capping and redistribution of membrane determinants.

THE EFFECTS OF dGuo AND dAdo IN IN VITRO MODEL SYSTEMS

From the data presented above dGuo and dAdo emerge as intoxi-

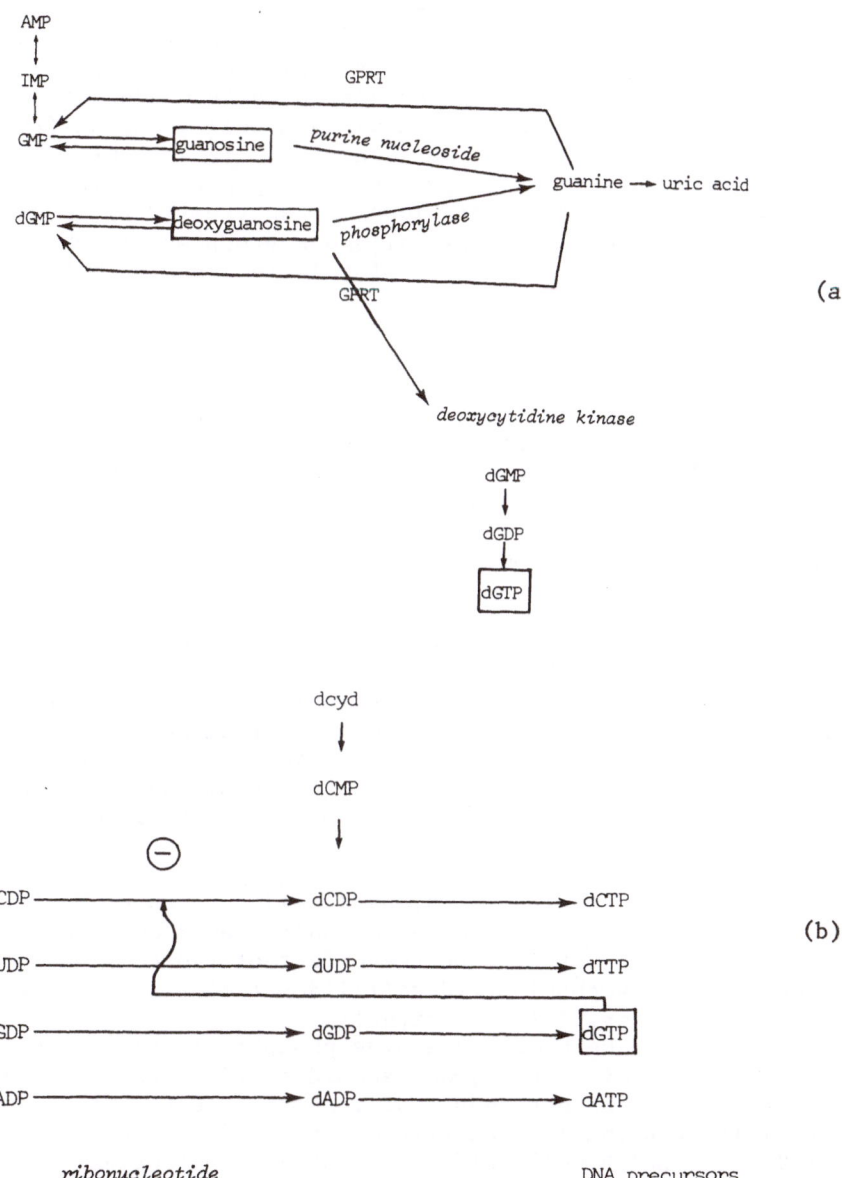

(a)

(b)

Fig. 1. PNP-deficiency: Pathophysiologic mechanism. (a) dGPT entrapment in lymphoid cells; (b) dGPT mediated inhibition of ribonucleotide reductase and the depletion of dCTP

cating compounds of the lymphoid system. As a consequence these
compounds are used in several model systems of T and B cell development and function. Several groups studied the effect of dGuo and
dAdo on the growth of human T and B cell lines either enzyme deficient or not (1). The substances also have been added to lymphocytes stimulated with either T cell or B cell mitogens (21,22,23)
and Gelfand et al. (24) and Heijnen et al. (25) studied the effect
on the T cell dependent antigen-specific plaque forming cell (PFC)
response of human peripheral blood lymphocytes (PBL). A different
approach was followed by e.g. Gelfand's group who incubated ADA⁻
precursor T cells on monolayers of cultured thymic epithelium either
ADA-deficient or not (26).

    A note of caution should accompany these approaches, since some
of the investigators used lymphocytes of normal donors to study the
effect of the compounds. The metabolic route of dAdo and dGuo in
ADA and PNP-containing cells, is different from the route in ADA⁻
and PNP⁻ cells. The results of these studies therefore do not necessarily reflect the condition of ADA- or PNP-deficiency.

    The results from these studies can be summarized as follows.
The observations of Gelfand et al. (26) with the thymic epithelial
model strongly suggest that ADA-deficiency (and probably also PNP-
deficiency) acts early in T cell differentiation. In addition
thymocytes appeared to be extremely sensitive for dGuo and dAdo,
actually they are more sensitive than T lymphocytes from peripheral
blood. This indicates that different developmental stages of T cells
show different sensitivities for dGuo and dAdo; this observation
correlates with the finding that the deoxynucleoside phosphorylating
capacity of thymocytes is high as compared to peripheral blood T
cells (27).

    Furthermore, peripheral blood T cells are more sensitive to
the toxic effects of the deoxy-compounds than B cells as could be
concluded from the studies on the effect of the compounds on established T and B lymphoblastoid cell lines (28). In contrast to this
difference in sensitivity, peripheral blood T cells and B cells
have about the same deoxynucleoside phosphorylating capacities (29).
To explain this discrepancy one should realize that the degree of
intoxication is the net result of formation, utilization and breakdown of the deoxynucleoside triphosphate. It has been suggested
that T cells and B cells differ in endo-5'-nucleotidase activity
in the sense that the entrapped triphosphates are more readily
broken down in B cells than in T cells. Finally it was shown (24,
25) that dGuo interferes with the in vitro induction of antigen-
specific suppressor cell function, whereas T helper function and
the differentiation of B cells into a PFC was unaffected. Heijnen
et al. (25) could show that the interference of dGuo with the suppressor cell circuit acts on the level of the T-precursor-suppressor
cell.

In PNP-deficient patients extremely high serum Ig-levels and even monoclonal Ig may occur, in addition to exaggerated specific antibody responses (9,11). This observation suggests imbalances in T cell mediated regulation of humoral immune responses. On the basis of the observations in the patients and the in vitro effects of dGuo on proliferation-dependent induction of antigen-specific suppressor cell function of normal peripheral blood lymphocytes, some authors did suggest that in PNP-deficiency suppressor T cell function is lacking. Clinically these patients would thus be prone to develop auto-antibodies and even auto-immune disease (9). However, when we tested the blood of our PNP-deficient patient for antigen-specific Ts-function we did not find any abnormalities (12). In addition, our patient did not (yet) develop auto-antibodies.

THERAPY IN ADA AND PNP-DEFICIENCY

In ADA⁻-SCID patients bone marrow transplantation is regarded as the therapy of choice. Indeed, several ADA⁻-SCID patients were successfully treated with (HLA-identical, MLC-negative) bone marrow. Most of them are clinically and immunologically completely normal. In some of them the bony abnormalities as well as the neurological abnormalities, as present before transplantation, had disappeared. As far as the metabolic abnormalities are concerned the engrafted cells are able to lower toxic Ado and dAdo levels in plasma and urine, which results in lowering of dATP of red cells and lymphocytes (30). However, the levels of these metabolites do not always become entirely normal but evidently low enough to endow the patient with an adequate immunological defense (31). Unfortunately, in most instances no suitable bone marrow donor is available for a patient with ADA⁻-SCID. Thus other therapeutic approaches have to be considered. Polmar et al. (32) were the first to show that transfusion of irradiated erythrocytes of normal donors may be beneficial to ADA⁻-SCID patients. The donor red cells deaminate accumulated Ado and dAdo and degrade them to purine bases and uric acid; plasma and urine Ado and dAdo decrease and dATP content of erythrocytes and lymphocytes is lowered subsequently. However, only 50% of ADA⁻-SCID patients seem to respond clinically and immunologically to enzyme replacement by repeated transfusion. Actually, those patients, having some residual immunological function before treatment, do respond and those having no demonstrable T or B cell function do not (33). Those patients that do not respond display nevertheless a decrease in toxic metabolites. This finding seems to challenge the concept that the clearing of the toxic metabolites is essential for a successful treatment. However, the lack of response in these patients can be explained in another way: chronic exposure to toxic metabolites may have resulted in either the loss of stem cells or pre-T cells or irreversible damage of thymic tissue as a result of involution by toxic dATP. This point of view offers additional therapeutic approaches, i.e. the administration of thymic factors

and transplantation of cultured thymic epithelium. Indeed,
Rubinstein et al. (34) showed that a patient with ADA⁻-SCID did not
improve on enzyme replacement alone or on administration of thymosin
alone; however, immunological reconstitution and clinical improvement could be achieved when both were combined.

In PNP-deficiency experience with repeated enzyme replacement
is restricted to two patients (12,35,36). Our own results of 5 years
of treatment can be summarized as follows: Enzyme replacement was
started when the patient was almost two years old; at the time the
T cell function as studied in vitro by measuring the proliferative
response to mitogens and allogeneic cells was completely negative (11). The transfusions consisted of 15 ml irradiated packed
red cells per kg bodyweight, given with a frequency of one transfusion in four weeks. The application of this regime of transfusion
enabled to maintain a subnormal PNP-activity of the circulating
erythrocytes (PNP-half-life of these erythrocytes is about 20-30
days). After each transfusion the nucleoside and deoxynucleoside
excretion decreases with concurrent rise of urinary uric acid excretion as well as a rise in serum uric acid. In addition the
dGTP-level of the erythrocytes decreased but did not become completely normal. Most importantly, also a change in the immunological
findings was observed, finally resulting in a partial and gradually
attained restoration of in vitro T cell function. Similar results
have been found in the Chicago-patient (36). The T cell function of
our patient never returned to normal during the past five years of
treatment with transfusion. Therefore, it is not surprising that
she still shows an excessive vulnerability for virus infections and
respiratory and skin infections do frequently occur. (Table 1 and
reference 12). Administration of deoxycytidine (dCyd) seems to be
a fourth potential therapeutic possibility in ADA and PNP deficiency. Administration of dCyd may bypass the enzyme ribonucleotide
reductase, thus restoring the synthesis of dCTP and subsequently
DNA-synthesis of the lymphocytes (Fig. 1). Already two years ago
dCyd was administered to a number of ADA⁻-patients and to our
patient with PNP-deficiency (35). However, neither orally, nor in-
travenously administered deoxycytidine (dosage 150 mg per kg/day)
has resulted in any patient in metabolic, immunologic or clinical
improvement. This could be explained by the degradation of the compound by cytidine deaminase in the mucosa of the gut or the liver.
Recently, we had the opportunity to treat our patient again with
dCyd, but now with concomitant treatment of the patient with an
inhibitor of the deaminase i.e. tetrahydrouridine (THU), which was
kindly supplied by Dr. C.Young, Sloan Kettering Institute. Treatment of the patient with subcutaneously administered THU (50 mg/kg
bodyweight/per day) followed by daily infusion of dCyd (50 mg/kg
bodyweight), was effective since dCyd was found in the urine. During
the monitoring of the immune status of the patient, it was found
that a substantial number (i.e. about 10%) of the freshly isolated
lymphocytes of the patient were in S-phase. This suggested that the

lymphocytes of the patients are hampered in vivo in the completion of the cellcycle. Most surprisingly, during dCyd/THU treatment the S-phase cells disappeared and the absolute number of lymphocytes concurrently increased (37). This suggests that the cells now were able to complete the cellcycle and that most probably in vivo lymphocyte proliferation has taken place. This observation seems directly to indicate the role of dCTP and the disturbance of lymphocytic DNA-synthesis in PNP-deficiency.

The molecular defects associated with an immune deficiency have added a new dimension to the knowledge of the function and organisation of the lymphoid system. It is to be expected that new molecular defects underlying immunodeficiency diseases will be unravelled in the near future. This may have an impact on the variety of therapeutic measures available.

REFERENCES

1. "Enzyme Defects and Immune Dysfunction", Ciba Symposium 68, Excerpta Medica, Amsterdam, pp. 1-289, (1979).
2. Martin, D.W., Jr., Gelfand, E.W., Ann. Rev. Biochem. 30:845-877 (1981).
3. Webster, A.D.B., Clin. Exp. Immunol. 49:1-10 (1982).
4. Cohen, A., Mansour, A., Dosch, H.M., Gelfand, E.W., Clin. Immunol. Immunopath. 15:245-250 (1980).
5. Bach, J.F., Imm. Today 2:225-227 (1981).
6. Cowan, M.J., Wara, D., Packman, S., Ammann, A.J., Yoshimo, M., Sweetman, L., Hijhan, W., Lancet 2:115-118 (1979).
7. Fisher, A., Munnich, A., Saudrebray, J.M., Mamas, S., Coude, F.X., Charpentier, C., Dray, F., Frézal, J., Griscelli, C., J. Clin. Immunol. 2:35-39 (1982).
8. Hirschhorn, R., Ciba Symposium 68, Excerpta Medica, Amsterdam, pp. 35-49 (1979).
9. Ammann, A., Ciba Symposium 68, Excerpta Medica, Amsterdam, pp. 55-69 (1979).
10. Stoop, J.W., Eijsvogel, V.P., Zegers, B.J.M., Blok-Schut, B., van Bekkum, D.W., Ballieux, R.E., Clin. Immunol. Immunopath. 6:289-298 (1976).
11. Stoop, J.W., Zegers, B.J.M., Hendrickx, G.F.M., Siegenbeek van Heukelom, L.H., Stall, G.E.J., de Bree, P.K., Wadman, S.K., Ballieux, R.E., N. Engl. J. Med. 296:651-655 (1977).
12. Stoop, J.W., Zegers, B.J.M., Kuis, W., Roord, J.J., Duran, M., Wadman, S.K., Staal, G.E.J., in: "Primary Immunodeficiencies", Seligmann, M., Hitzig, W.H. (eds.), Elsevier, pp. 301-311 (1980).
13. Watson, A.R., Evans, D.L.K., Mauden, H.B., Miller, V., Rogers, P.A., Arch. Disease of Childhood 56:563-565 (1981).
14. Zabay, J.M., de la Concha, E.G., Pascual-Salcedo, D., Subiza, J.L., Lozano, C., Bootello, A., 5th Eur. Immunol. Meeting (1982).

15. Cohen, A., Gudas, L.J., Ulman, B., Martin, D.W., Jr., Ciba
    Symposium 68, Excerpta Medica, Amsterdam, pp. 101-109,
    (1979).
16. Watson, A.R., Simmonds, H.A., Webster, D.R., Layward, L.,
    Evans, D.I.K., J. Clin. Chem and Biochem. 20:431 (1982).
17. Carson, D.A., Kaye, J., Seegmiller, J.E., Proc. Natl. Acad. Sci.
    USA 74:5677-5681 (1977).
18. Kefford, R.M., Fox, R.M., Cancer Res. 42:324-330 (1982).
19. Carson, D.A., Wasson, D.B., Lakow, E., Kamatani, N., Proc. Natl.
    Acad. Sci. USA 79:3438-3852 (1982).
20. Hershfield, M.S., Kredich, N.M., Ownby, D.R., Ownby, H.,
    Buckley, R., J. Clin. Invest. 63:807-811 (1979).
21. Ochs, U.H., Chen, S.H., Ochs, H.D. Osborne, W.R., Scott, C.R.
    J. Immunol. 22:2424-2429 (1979).
22. Hayward, A.R., Clin. Exp. Immunol. 41:141-149 (1980).
23. Spaapen, L.J.M., Dane, M.E., Toebes, E., Tepas, B., Staal,
    G.E.J., Duran, M., Kuis, W., Rijkers, G.T., Zegers, B.J.M.,
    Adv. Exp. Med. Biol. (in press).
24. Gelfand, E.W., Lee, J.J., Dosch, H.M., Proc. Natl. Acad. Sci.
    USA 76:1998-2002 (1979).
25. Heijnen, C.J., UytdeHaag, F., Pot, K.H., Ballieux, R.E., in:
    "Human B-lymphocyte Function: Activation and Immunoregulation",
    Fauci, A.S., Ballieux, R.E. (eds.), Raven Press, pp. 239-253
    (1982).
26. Shore, A., Dosch, H.M., Galfand, E.W., Clin. Exp. Immunol.
    44:152-155 (1981).
27. Cohen, A., Lee, J.W.W., Dosch, H.M., Gelfand, E.W., J. Immunol.
    125:1578-1582 (1980).
28. Mitchell, B., Mejias, E., Daddona, P., Kelley, W.N., Proc. Natl.
    Acad. Sci. USA 75:5011-5014 (1978).
29. North, M.E., Newton, C.A., Webster, A.D.B., Clin. Exp. Immunol.
    42:523-529 (1980).
30. Hirshhorn, R., Roegner-Maniscalco, V., Kuritsky, L., Rosen,
    F.S., 68, 1387-1393 (1981).
31. Chen, S.H., Ochs, H.D., Scott, C.R., Giblett, E.R., Tingle,
    A.J., J. Clin. Invest. 62:1386-1389 (1978).
32. Polmar, S.H., Stern, R.C., Schwartz, A.L., Wetzler, E.M.,
    Chase, P.A., Hirschhorn, R., N. Engl. J. Med. 195:1337-1343
    (1976).
33. Polmar, S.H., in: "Inborn Errors of Specific Immunity",
    Pollara, B., Pickering, K.J., Meuwissen, H.J., Porter, I.H.
    (eds.), Academic Press, New York, pp. 341-351 (1979).
34. Rubinstein, A., Hirschhorn, R., Sicklick, M., Murphy, R.A.,
    N. Engl. J. Med. 300:387-392 (1979).
35. Zegers, B.J.M., Stoop, J.W., Staal, G.E.J., Wadman, S.K.,
    Ciba Symposium 68, Excerpta Medica, Amsterdam, pp. 231-247
    (1979).
36. Rich, K.C., Mejias, E., Fox, I.H., N. Engl. J. Med. 303:973-977
    (1980).

37. Rijkers, G.T., Zegers, B.J.M., Spaapen, L.J.M., Rutgers, D.H., Kuis, W., Roord, J.J., Stoop, J.W., Adv. Exp. Med. Biol. (in press).

IMMUNOLOGICALLY DISTINCT FORMS OF PRIMARY HYPERGAMMAGLOBULINAEMIA:

STUDIES USING POKEWEED MITOGEN AND EPSTEIN-BARR VIRUS

T.A.E. Platts-Mills[*], R.S. Pereira, A.D.B. Webster
and S.R. Wilkins

Division of Immunology, Clinical Research Centre
Harrow, Middlesex, England

Since the first demonstration that some patients with repeated
attacks of respiratory tract infection lacked serum immunoglobulins,
there have been many attempts to understand the immunological basis
for this deficiency. Some of the patients present with infections
within the first year of life and many of these show an X-linked
pattern of inheritance, X-linked agammaglobulinaemia or XLA. The
boys and young men with XLA are in many ways distinct from the patients who present after the age of 2 years who show no sex bias and
usually no family history; common variable immune deficiency or
CVID. There are also a few cases where hypogammaglobulinaemia is
associated with the presence of a thymoma, these cases generally
present over the age of 45 years and they have a much worse prognosis. The investigation of all these patients has changed progressive-
ly over the last 10 years in parallel with advances in our general
understanding of antibody production.

When the distinction between T cell and B cells became clear it
seemed likely that these patients would lack B cells or have abnormal B cells. In keeping with this, it was found that their lymph
nodes lacked germinal centres, and completely lacked plasma cells.
However, when it became possible to identify B cells directly by
visualizing the Ig on their surface (SmIg), many patients with CVID
were found with normal or near normal numbers of circulating

[*] Current address:
 Division of Allergy and Clinical Immunology, Box 225, Department
 of Medicine, University of Virginia, Charlottesville, Virginia
 22908, U.S.A.

B cells (1). This was not true for patients with XLA who had no detectable B cells and similarly the patients with thymoma had few or
no circulating B cells. Soon after this time animal data began to
accumulate suggesting that T cells could not only help antibody production but could also suppress it. In 1974 Waldmann and his colleagues found evidence that lymphocytes from some of their patients
with CVID showed abnormal suppressor activity in vitro (2). Subsequently, other groups found similar evidence but a true abnormality
of in vitro T cell activity was found to be present in less than
one-fifth of the patients (3). Interestingly, the groups of patients
who most consistently showed abnormal suppressor T cell activity
were the patients with a thymoma (4-7).

    The demonstration of functional defects of T cells has been
largely dependent on the use of pokeweed mitogen to stimulate Ig
production in vitro. Pokeweed mitogen (PWM) is strictly T dependent (8-10), and is unaffected by whether the T cells and B cells are
autologous or allogeneic. Using purified B cells (or non T cells)
it is possible to test the helper activity of a patient's T cells:
using a mixture of normal B cell and normal T cells, it is possible
to test a patient's T cells for abnormal suppressor activity (7).
Simply mixing the mononuclear cells of a patient with normal mononuclear cells may give very confusing results because normal T cells
can suppress Ig production if they are present in a high ratio relative to functional B cells (3,11). This is particularly relevant
in relation to hypogammaglobulinaemia because some of the patients
have reduced numbers of B cells or B cells which may not "contribute"
to T cell: B cell ratios (12). Using techniques in which the numbers
of B cells and T cells in a culture are carefully controlled, it
appears that the majority of patients with CVID and XLA have T cells
which function fully normally in vitro. Furthermore, in most cases
these T cells show normal T cell markers using OKT monoclonal antibodies (13,14).

    Early in the investigation of hypogammaglobulinaemia it was
clear that most of the patients had normal delayed hypersensitivity
(DH) to recall antigens (15). In keeping with this, most of the
patients do not suffer from diseases associated with T cell deficiency. It is worth pointing out that profound abnormalities of T
cell help or increased suppression in the PWM system can be present
in patients who have apparently normal DH. The severely depressed
T cell numbers and T cell proliferative responses to PHA, which are
a diagnostic feature of babies with SCID and that occur in homo-
sexuals with severe immune deficiency (16), are not seen in cases
of chronic late onset hypogammaglobulinaemia or XLA. Having said
this, we have recently seen a patient with thymoma and hypogammaglobulinaemia who developed deficiency of both eosinophils and
basophils. This is interesting for two reasons. Firstly, because
these cells are thought to be essential for cutaneous basophil
hypersensitivity (CBH) and CBH is thought to play an important role

in cellular immunity including not only parasite rejection but also tumour rejection (17). Secondly, since patients had a marked increase in activated suppressor T cells, it seems possible that these T cells influenced the production of B cells, eosinophils and basophils in vivo (18). Thus it is possible that prolonged presence of activated suppressor cells (i.e. many years) may lead to progressive deterioration of cellular immunity as humoral immunity and may contribute to the poor prognosis of these patients.

In early experiments on B cells from patients with CVID, it was found that PWM would induce some cells to transform into plasma cells (1). Using quantitative assays the quantities of Ig secreted were generally very low (2,3), and even under optimal conditions the quantities of IgG or IgA relative to IgM were always very low (12). It was also clear from those studies that the minority of patients with abnormal suppressor T cell activity had very few circulating B cells and that they could not be induced to produce Ig in vitro using PWM (12). Recently, using Epstein-Barr virus (EBV) to activate Ig production in cultures of T depleted mononuclear cells, we have been able to re-examine the results obtained using PWM (13). Using EBV, cells from most patients with CVID will produce normal quantities of IgM and IgD with very little IgG or IgA. This pattern was very similar to that seen with cord blood or fetal liver B cells. These observations led to the conclusion that the B cells circulating in the patients with CVID were probably normal immature B cells and that they were probably present in normal numbers. By contrast, cells from patients with XLA failed to respond to EBV or responded late and produced limited quantities of IgM with surprising quantities of IgD (13). Results on patients with abnormal suppressor T cell activity with or without thymoma again confirmed the difference of this group from the other patients with CVID, in that they produced IgG in near normal quantities with or without IgM. It appears that this group of patients have a small number of circulating B cells but that these few cells are probably "mature" in type.

In conclusion, it is now possible to assess the function of peripheral blood B cells and T cells from patients with hypogammaglobulinaemia using reliable techniques. The results suggest that several different mechanisms are involved. In the boys with XLA there appears to be a failure of B cell production by the bone marrow, so that pre B cells, immature B cells and mature B cells are all lacking. In most of these cases T cells are normal. In the "late onset" patients who have normal numbers of SmIgM+ve cells, these cells appear to be "immature" and comparable to those found in cord blood. The acquired defect in these patients is probably in the mechanism or micro environment in which antigen is presented to B cells or alternatively in the mechanism by which immature B cells respond to antigen. Again, in most of these patients, T cells are apparently normal. Finally, there is a small group of patients, including those with a thymoma, who have circulating activated suppressor T cells and in whom T cells may well be responsible for the failure of B cell (and eosinophil) production. The presence of a few circulating mature B cells in these patients supports the view that the suppressor cells act preferentially on bone marrow pre B cells or other precursors of immature B cells.

REFERENCES

1. Wu, L.Y., Lawton, A.R. and Cooper, M.D., J. Clin. Invest. 52:3180–3189 (1973).
2. Waldmann, T.A., Durm, M., Broder, S., Blackman, M., Blaese, R.M. and Strober, W., Lancet ii:609–613 (1974).
3. de la Concha, E.G., Oldham, G., Webster, A.D.B., Asherson, G.L. and Platts-Mills, T.A.E., Clin. Exp. Immunol. 27:208–215 (1977).
4. Waldmann, T.A., Broder, S., Durm, M., Blackman, M., Krakauer, R. and Meade, B., Trans. Assoc. Am. Physicians 88:120 (1975).
5. Moretta, L., Mingari, M.C., Webb, S.R., Pearl, E.R., Lydyard, P.M., Grossi, C.E., Lawton, A.R. and Cooper, M.D., Eur. J. Immunol. 7:696–700 (1977).
6. Litwin, S.D. and Zanjani, E.D., Nature 266:57–59 (1977).
7. Platts-Mills, T.A.E., de Gast, G.C., Webster, A.D.B., Asherson, G.L. and Wilkins, S.R., Clin. Exp. Immunol. 44:383:388 (1981).
8. Janossy, G. and Greaves, M., Immunol. Rev. 24:177–191 (1975).
9. Keightley, R.G., Cooper, M.D. and Lawton, A.R., J. Immunol. 117:1538 (1976).
10. Janossy, G., de la Concha, G., Luquetti, A., Snajdr, M.J., Waxdal, M.J. and Platts-Mills, T.A.E., Scand. J. Immunol. 6:109–123 (1977).
11. Gmelig-Meyling, F., Uytdehaag, A.G. and Ballieux, R.E., Cell. Immunol. 33:156–169 (1977).
12. de Gast, G.C., Wilkins, S.R., Webster, A.D.B., Rickinson, A. and Platts-Mills, T.A.E., Clin. Exp. Immunol. 42:535–544 (1980).
13. Pereira, R.S., Webster, A.D.B. and Platts-Mills, T.A.E., Eur. J. Immunol. 12:540–546 (1982).
14. Pereira, R.S. and Platts-Mills, T.A.E., in: "Clinics in Haematology", 11:3, G. Janossy, Ed., W.B. Saunders Co. Ltd. pp. 589–605 (1982).
15. Asherson, G.L. and Webster, A.D.B., "Diagnosis and treatment of immune deficiency diseases, Blackwell, Oxford (1980).
16. Gottlieb, M.R., Schroff, R., Schanker, H.M., Weisman, J.D., Peng Phim Fan, Wolff, R.A. and Saxon, A., N. Engl. J. Med. 305:1425–1431 (1981).
17. Askenase, P., J. Allergy Clin. Immunol. 64:79–89 (1979).
18. Mitchell, E.B., Chapman, M.D., Pope, F.M., Crow, J., Jouhal, S.S. and Platts-Mills, Lancet i:127–129 (1982).

T CELL SUBSET RESPONSES IN VARIED IMMUNODEFICIENCY SYNDROMES

F. Caballero, P. Kohler and A.R. Hayward

Departments of Pediatrics and Medicine
University of Colorado Health Sciences Center
Denver, Colorado 80262, U.S.A.

INTRODUCTION

Patients with common varied immunodeficiency syndromes (CVID) are heterogeneous as regards the number and function of T cells in their blood (1,2). A minority of CVID patients has strong suppressor activity in in vitro functional tests and many have a relative increase of cells in blood which bear the suppressor-cytotoxic phenotype, T8[+] (3). A primary increase in suppressor cells may contribute to hypogammaglobulinemia in some patients with thymoma (4) but in the majority of CVID patients it is unclear whether the increase in T8[+] cells is primary or whether it results from antigen stimulation. We therefore examined the possibility that antigen stimulation might maintain increased numbers or proportions of T8[+] cells in CVID patients by determining the phenotype of their T cell blasts in cultures stimulated with tetanus toxoid. The rationale for this approach derives from the observation that soluble antigens normally elicit proliferation by T4[+] cells while cell-associated antigens (such as allogenic cells) elicit responses by both T4[+] and T8[+] cells.

METHODS

Blood from patients and healthy controls was defibrinated and centrifuged so that the serum could be recovered for medium supplementation. Mononuclear cells (MNC) were separated on Ficoll-Hypaque gradients, washed twice and adjusted to 10^6/ml in RPM1 1640 with gentamicin and 10% autologous serum. Cultures were in 20 ml volumes in Lux (Cat. #5350) tissue culture flasks with 2 Lf of tetanus toxoid antigen (given by Wyeth Labs) per ml. They were incubated for 6 days in a 5% CO_2 atmosphere; then the blasts were recovered from the 40%

167

interface of a discontinuous Percoll gradient. The cells were stained
with monoclonal antibodies and fluorescein-conjugated goat-anti-mouse
IgG (Cappel Labs) as before (5).

In certain experiments the cultures were reduced to 1 ml volumes
on the 6th day and pulsed for 2 hours with 5 uCi of tritiated thymidine (TRA 61 Amersham Searle). Viable cells were recovered from a
Ficoll Hypaque gradient and incubated with monoclonal antibodies as
above. After washing in Hanks BSS with 0.1% BSA and 0.1% sodium azide
they were placed in the wells of Falcon 3912 flexible assay plates
which had been precoated with affinity-purified goat-anti-mouse IgG
(Tago). The cells were allowed to become adhered during 30 minutes
incubation at 37°; non-adherent cells were then flushed away with a
stream of cold Hanks and 0.1 mls of 0.1% SDS was added to the wells
to lyse the adherent cells. The plates were cut up and wells, with
cell lysates, were tranferred to counting vials with aqueous counting
solution for liquid scintillation counting.

RESULTS

Thirteen patients and seven controls were studied. No T cell
blasts were obtained from two of the patients and one of the controls
and these individuals are excluded from the analysis. The cells recovered from the Percoll gradients from the remaining individuals
comprised over 66% cells with large, blast, morphology and in most
preparations about 80% of the cells were blasts. The subsets of
these cells as determined by immunofluorescence is shown in Fig. 1.
Four of the patients lie outside the range of the controls for
percent T8$^+$ blasts. To confirm that the cells we isolated and identified as T cell blasts were indeed dividing we measured the uptake
of tritiated thymidine by cells from two patients (one with increased T8$^+$ blasts) and one control. The results (Table 1) indicate
that T8$^+$ cells separated from the appropriate patient's blood had
incorporated thymidine.

Table 2 gives the T cell subset data on the patients' blood
mononuclear cells before culture, together with partinant clinical
data.

DISCUSSION

Our results suggest that the T8$^+$ cells of certain patients with
CVID acquire the buoyant density and morphology of blasts following
in vitro stimulation with Tetanus toxoid antigen. Confirmation that
the T8$^+$ blasts were dividing was obtained in one case by demonstrating uptake of tritiated thymidine. Only 4 of the 11 patients studied
had increased proportions of T8$^+$ blasts and this was accompanied by

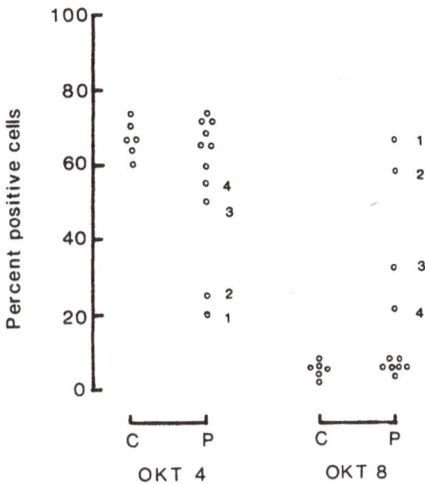

Fig. 1. Phenotype of T cell blasts from Tetanus toxoid stimulated cultures of controls (C) and common varied hypogammaglobulinemic patients (P) lymphocytes. The numbered results refer to patients identified in Table 2.

Table 1. Thymidine uptake by Tetanus toxoid-stimulated T cells of CVID patients

| | cmp of cells adhered with | |
	OKT 4	OKT 8
Patient 1	820	1900
Patient 6	2600	210
Controls	2916±300	175±55

reduced proportions of T4+ blasts. These 4 patients were not clearly separable from the remaining patients by clinical or laboratory criteria. Possible explanations for their increased response by T8+ cells include (1) that it results from a primary abnormality of T cell regulation or (2) that it is secondary to the patients' antibody deficiency. The variability between patients of the number of T8+ cells in their blood argues against a primary abnormality of T cell regulation and we consider that secondary changes are as likely. T cells generally respond to antigen in association with an HLA antigen which is called the restriction antigen. In the case of T4+ cells the restriction antigens belong to the HLA-DR series while for T8+ cells they belong to HLA A, B or C. Suppressor cells appear capable of binding to antigen in the absence of any restricting an-

Table 2.   T cell subset data on the patients' blood mononuclear
           cells before culture

Patient	Age (yrs.)	Sex	Serum immunoglobulins[†]			Blood lymphocyte subsets[††]			
			IgG	IgA	IgM	T3	T4	T8	SIg[†]
1	62	F	188	13	36	61	36	21	8
2	60	M	177	9	59	64	27	36	4
3	33	F	8	10	35	68	33	32	7
4	22	F	4	1	14	71	33	35	9

[†] As mg/dL
[††] As percent of Ficoll-Hypaque separated MNC

tigen. Antigen presentation to helper T cells is through HLA-DR
bearing cells of the mononuclear phagocyte series so that, in the
absence of antibody, more antigen will remain free and might con-
ceivably stimulate suppressor cells. In antibody deficient patients
this might result in an expansion of suppressor cell clones so that
these cells would dominate a response in vitro. If this view were
correct one might expect to find differences in the subset distribution of responder T cells in patients' blood depending on the antigen
used to elicit a response. Dietary antigens, which are known to
elicit suppressor responses in mice (6), might be particularly effective inducers of suppressor responses in some immunodeficiencies
because of their increased amounts in patients' sera (7).

ACKNOWLEDGEMENT

Partly supported by grants HD 13733 and RR 69 from the NIH.

REFERENCES

1. Webster, A.D.B. and Asherson, G.L., Clin. Exp. Immunol. 18:449
    (1974).
2. Geha, R.S., Schneeberger, E., Mesler, E. and Rosen, F.S.,
    New Engl. J. Med. 291:1 (1974).
3. Reinherz, E.L., Cooper, M.D., Schlossman, S.F. and Rosen, R.S.,
    J. Clin. Invest. 68:699 (1981).
4. Hayward, A.R. and Kurnick, J.T., J. Immunol. 126:50 (1981).
5. Hayward, A.R., Paolucci, P., Webster, A.D.B. and Kohler, P.F.,
    Clin. Exp. Immunol. (1982) (in press).

6. Challacombe, S.J. and Tomasi, T.B., J. Exp. Med. 152:1459
    (1980).
7. Cunningham-Rundles, C., Brandeis, W.E., Good, R.A. and Day,
    N.K., J. Clin. Invest. 64:272 (1979).

IMMUNE DYSFUNCTIONS IN ATAXIA-TELANGIECTASIA

A.I. Berkel, F. Ersoy, Ö. Sanal, G. Ciliv, O. Yeğin

Hacettepe University, Institute of Child Health
Immunology Unit and Biochemistry Department
Ankara, Turkey

Ataxia-telangiectasia (AT) is an autosomal recessive immunodeficiency, characterized by progressive ataxia, oculocutaneous te-
langiectasia, recurrent sinopulmonary infections, absent or reduced
serum IgA, low serum IgE and decreased or undetectable IgG2, deficiency of cellular immunity and various endocrine disorders. Elevated serum alpha fetoprotein, chromosomal abnormalities and defective DNA repair following X irradiation or after incubation of lymphocytes with mutagens are other abnormal findings in AT. A high
incidence of malignancies, particularly lymphoreticular types, has
also been reported (1,2). With the recent demonstration of a clasto-
genic factor, prenatal diagnosis of AT became possible (3) but the
etiopathogenesis is still unknown. The major goals in the research
of patients with AT include reliable identification of carriers or
heterozygotes, differentiation of any heterogeneity within the group
of A-T patients and identification of pathognomonic laboratory findings which would confirm early diagnosis.

Since 1968, we have been interested in AT and 112 patients from
87 families have registered in the Immunology Unit of Hacettepe
Children's Hospital. High incidence of cousin marriages or inbreed-
ing in Turkey and referrals of many patients to our Center are the
major factors influencing the number of AT cases seen by our group.

In this presentation the immune dysfunctions and abnormalities
observed in our AT patients will be summarized. I would like to
acknowledge the collaborations of Drs. G. Klein, M.C. Masucci,
G. Masucci of the Karolinska Institute and Drs. Werner and Gertrude
Henle of the Philadelphia Children's Hospital.

Table 1.   Delayed Hypersensitivity (Skin tests)

	A-T Patients		Controls[*]	
	no. positives no. tested	%	no. positives no. tested	%
PHA	64/77	83.1	113/167	61.6
CANDIDA	21/82	25.6	49/126	38.9
SKSD	45/83	54.2	79/131	60.3
PPD	11/78	14.1	31/103	30.0

* age range 5-16 years.

CELL MEDIATED IMMUNITY

Cell mediated immunity was assessed by various laboratory tests. Absolute lymphocyte count was checked in 90 AT cases. The mean was $2303/\mu l$, the range was $806-6032/\mu l$. 39 patients (43.3%) had values $<2000/\mu l$, in 7 patients (7.7%) the counts were $<1000/\mu l$.

Skin test responses are summarized in Table 1. There were significant differences in responses for the candida and PPD antigens when compared with healthy controls.

Examination of lymphocyte subpopulations showed significant decrease in E rosettes and $Ea\mu$ rosettes and significant increase in $EA\gamma$ rosettes (Table 2). We found that suppressor cells to be increased when detected by monoclonal antisera. OKT4/OKT8 (helper/suppressor) ratio was less than 1 in 8 out of 16 patients tested.

Natural killer (NK) cell activity was studied by using two different targets, namely K562 and Daudi cells. AT patients' lymphocytes showed good cytotoxicity with K562 cells before and after incubation with interferon (Fig. 1-3). The cytotoxicity with Daudi cells was not as good as that observed with K562. Again interferon incubation increased cytotoxicity (Fig. 4-6). We studied lymphotoxin production in 11 AT patients by using different doses of PHA (Fig. 7). Lymphotoxin production was normal in 5. Three of these had abnormal blastogenic transformation whereas the other two had normal in vitro blastogenic response to PHA. Of 6 patients with abnormal lymphotoxin production, 5 had low blastogenic response.

Neutrophil chemotaxis was found to be normal in 10 AT patients when compared with 22 age matched healthy controls. However random migration was found to be increased in AT cases. Chemotactic index

Table 2. Lymphocyte Subpopulations

	A-T Patients	Controls
E rosettes (%)	56.7±11.0[*] (34–72)[**] n=20[+]	69.2±8.0 P<0.01 (53–75) n=79
EA rosettes (EAγ) (%)	18.5±7.9 (5–36) n=19	12.25±5.56 P<0.01 (4–22) n=33
EAC rosettes (%)	22.2±12.76 (11–56) n=17	17.75±6.16 P> 0.05 (11–56) n=33
EAμ rosettes (%)	8.2±3.73 (5–16) n=10	15.44±2.6 P<0.01 (6–33) n=10
B lymphocytes (%) (S Ig, Poly-Val.)	17.6±7.06 (10–29) n=10	14.63±4.20 P>0.05 (7–23) n=22

* mean ± 1 S.D.
** Range
+ number examined

Table 3. Blastic Transformation

	no. responders[*] no. tested	% responding	Stimulation index mean	range
PHA	28/60	46.6	73.8	0.97–235
CANDIDA	17/51	33.3	5.0	0.64–64.9
SKSD	8/45	17.8	3.5	0.76–56.2
MLC	15/25	60.0		

* responder: PHA-SI>20
            CAND-SI>2.5
            SKSD-SI>2.5

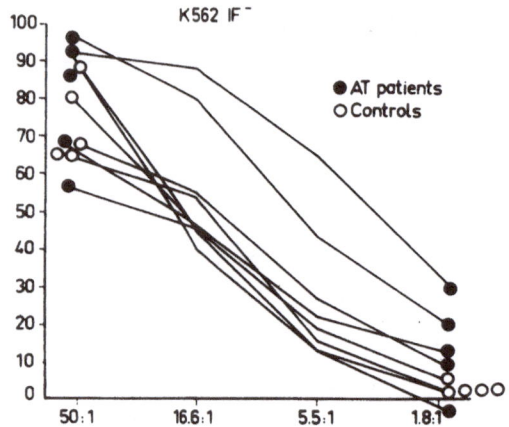

Fig. 1.   Cytotoxicity against K562 cells before incubation with
          interferon (Abscissa shows effector cell/target cell ratio).

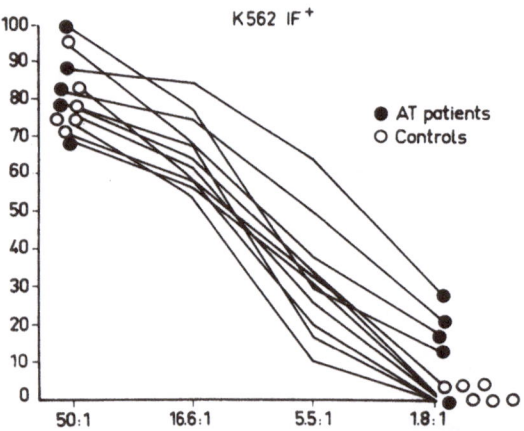

Fig. 2.   Cytotoxicity against K562 cells after incubation with
          interferon (Abscissa shows effector cell/target cell ratio).

and chemotactic difference parameters were significantly lower in
AT patients (Fig. 8). These lower values might be due to increased
random migration. No correlation between increased susceptibility
to infection and chemotaxis values could be observed. Serim IgA was
low in 4 patients. IgA values and chemotaxis results also did not
show any correlation.

In vitro blastic transformation responses to PHA, Candida SKSD
and allogeneic lymphocytes are seen in Table 3. Fourty six percent
of cases responded to PHA, and 60% had MLC response. Response to

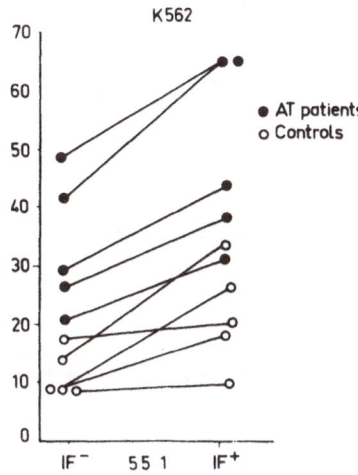

Fig. 3. Cytotoxicity against K562 cells before and after incubation
with interferon at an effector cell target cell ratio of
5.5:1

Candida and SKSD antigens were lower with respective values of 33%
and 17.8%. We found that AT serum to be inhibitory for the in vitro
PHA response in more than 40% of the patients.

HUMORAL IMMUNITY

Table 4 shows serum immunoglobulin levels. IgA deficiency was
observed in 38 percent of cases. As it is well known it varies
between 30% and 70% in different series in the literature.

Table 4. Serum Immunoglobulins (mg/dl)

	no. tested	mean±S.D.	range	low	percent
IgA	97	72.5±57.5	0-300	37/97	38%
IgG	98	971.6±390	75-1810	1/98	
IgM	98	157.7±62.4	15-360	1/98	
IgE*	29	18.4±22.5	0-73.9	23/29	79%

* presented as U/ml, normal value is 25 U/ml.

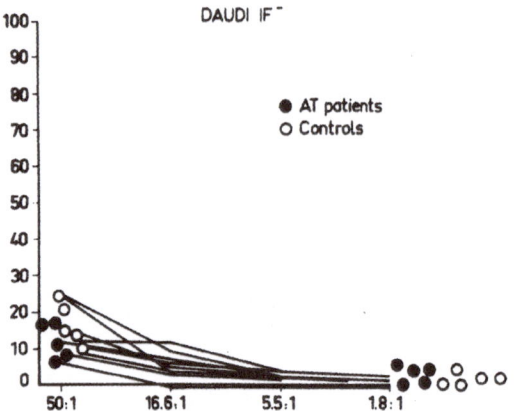

Fig. 4. Cytotoxicity against Daudi cells before incubation with
         interferon (Abscissa shows effector cell/target cell ratio).

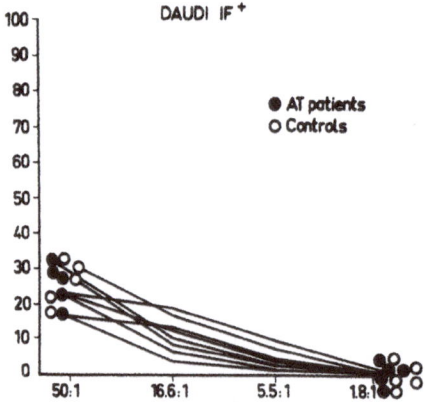

Fig. 5. Cytotoxicity against Daudi cells after incubation with
         interferon (Abscissa shows effector cell/target cell ratio).

     Serum IgE was low in 23 out of 29 patients (79%) and there was
association of low IgA and low IgE in 7 patients.

     IgG subgroups were studied with the collaboration of Drs. Vivian
Oxelius and Lars Hanson in 22 patients and IgG2 was very low or undetectable in all 22 patients studied (4).

     Ten of these had IgA deficiency. In 5 it was not demonstrable
(<0.01gL), in another 5 IgG2 was very low. In the remaining 12, IgG2
levels were low or in the lower range. There was no difference be-

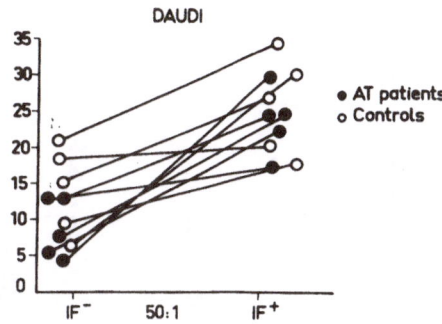

Fig. 6.   Cytotoxicity against Daudi cells, before and after incubation with interferon at an effector cell/target cell ratio
of 50:1.

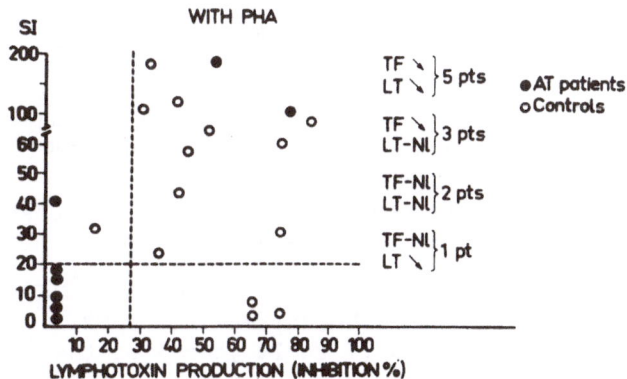

Fig. 7.   Lymphotoxin production with PHA [Abscissa shows percent
inhibition, ordinate shows stimulation index (SI)]
TF: Blastic transformation, LT: Lymphotoxin production
Dotted lines indicate normal values

tween patients with low and normal IgA levels. IgG1 was increased
in 9 patients and 8 had levels above the age related mean (P<0.001).
IgG3 was increased in 2 patients and 12 had levels above the age related mean. IgG4 was undetectable in all but 3 patients (0.01 to
0.06g/L). Nine patients with undetectable or low IgG2 including 4
with IgA deficiency and 5 without it, had chronic lung disease or
chronic sinusitis or both. The remaining 8 patients in the group

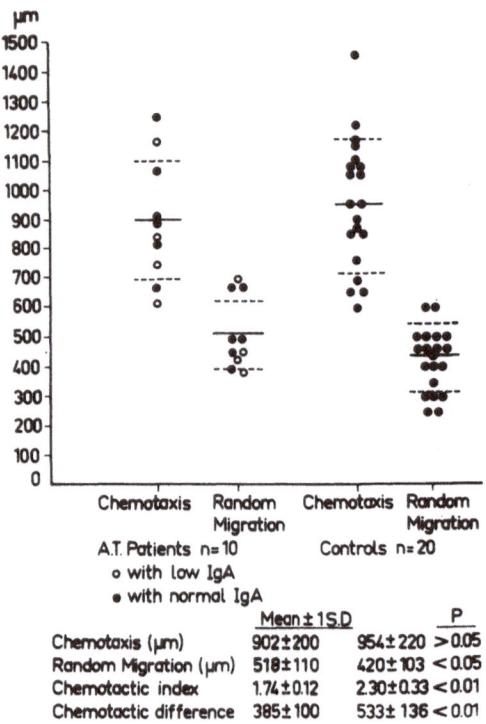

Fig. 8. Neutrophil chemotaxis and random migration in A-T
         patients and controls.

with chronic infections had borderline low IgG2 levels (3 with IgA
deficiency). Four patients (7 to 13 years) of the 5 without history
of frequent infections had normal IgA levels (0.78 to 2.04g/L) and
had IgG2 levels one of the highest noted in this study (1.30 to
1.67g/L). The 5 th patient had low IgA (0.15g/L) and very low IgG2
levels, but he was only 19 months old (4).

     Now I will present antibody response to EBV in AT patients. We
studied 27 AT patients, 22 of their parents, 23 healthy controls,
other immunodeficiency diseases and their family members. Anti-VCA
antibodies were present in all AT patients. The titers were increased
(>1:320) in 55.6% of cases; 48.2 percent of the patients had increased titers to early antigen (EA). Antibodies to the EBV associated nuclear antigen (EBNA) was low in 44.2% of the patients. The
geometric means of anti-VCA were 3 to 4 fold higher and anti-EBNA
six-fold lower than those of the control groups (5). AT patients
with low anti-EBNA titers tended to have more advanced T cell deficiencies than AT patients with moderate anti-EBNA titers as detected by total lymphocyte and T lymphocyte count and skin test responses.

Table 5. Adenosine Deaminase (ADA) and Nucleoside Phosphorlylase (NP)

	RED CELLS		LYMPHOCYTES	
	ADA[*]	NP[**]	ADA[+]	NP[++]
CONTROLS	55.6±18.5 (31.1-98.3) n=23	37.76±13.4 (13.1 -114.2) n=23	1.22±1.15 (0.38-5.33) n=20	1.17±0.10 (0.32-4.0) n=19
A-T	56.8±10.9 (41.5-87.0) n=12	34.7 ±11.5 (14.1 - 79.9) n=12	1.44±1.16 (0.51-3.89) n=7	1.41±0.18 (0.19-5.49) n=7

[*]   micromol uric acid/hr/gHb
[**] micromol uric acid/min/gHb
[+]   micromol uric acid/hr/mg protein
[++] micromol uric acid/min/mg protein
    Figures in pranthesis represent the range

The results support the hypothesis that a functioning T cell system is required to release EBNA from EBV genome carrying cells for initial maintained production of anti EBNA (5).

Our studies of adenosine deaminase (ADA) and nucleoside phosphorylase (NP) in red cells and lymphocytes in AT patients showed no significant differences from the healthy controls (Table 5).

AFP is reported to be increased in AT patients and high levels are claimed to be a marker for the disease (6). Our experience with 42 AT patients revealed that serum AFP is not increased in all cases and 11 of them exhibited normal levels. Determinations were done by RIA and repeated twice. The results were confirmed at the NIH at Dr. Waldmann's laboratory.

I would like to mention that ADP ribose polymerase activity in lymphocytes from 5 AT cases did not differ from the healthy controls. However, after exposure to 500 rad. irradiation, increase in that enzyme activity was less in the patients (0,2,9,12,25%) than the control group (30,36,37,38,39%).

Various chromosome abnormalities such as breaks, endoreduplications, rearrangements, etc. are reported in AT patient (7,8). We studied 24 AT patients, but the chromosome cultures grew successfully in only 16. Karyograms of 13 showed increase in breaks and rearrangements. 3 patients had 14q translocation.

Finally, I would like to mention the results of a recent study carried out on 12 AT patients from 8 families by Gatti and coworkers at Los Angeles (8). They found decreased T cells, elevated B cells, decreased PHA responses, variable suppressor cell activity and decreased serum IgA and IgG2. AFP in serum was elevated. Thymosin α_1 levels were not different than those of the controls. The following parameters relating to cell membrane and cytoskeletal functions were abnormal: Increased Con A capping, increased cyclic nucleotides (cAMP and cGMP) of lymphocytes and decreased chemotactic response of neutrophils. With these data they suggested that a cytoskeletal defect (either primary or secondary) may underline the various abnormalities seen in AT.

In summary, we would like to restress that AT is a heterogenous disorder with numerous dysfunctions in cellular and humoral immunity. Several hypotheses such as an immunoregulatory defect, a hypophyseal defect, a defect in DNA repair and/or replication and a defect of cytoskeletal and microtubular integrity should be explored by using appropriate genetic, biochemical and immunological methods.

REFERENCES

1. Boder, E., in: "Immunodeficiency in man and animals", Sunderland Mass. Sinaeur Associates, pp. 255-270 (1975).
2. Yount, W.J., New Engl. J. Med. 306:541-543 (1982).
3. Shaham, M., Vass, R., Becker, Y., Yarkoni, S., Ornoy, A. and Kohn, G., J. Pediatr. 100:134-137 (1982).
4. Oxelius, V.A., Berkel, A.I. and Hanson, L.A., New Engl. J. Med. 306:515-517 (1982).
5. Berkel, A.I., Henle, W., Hanle, G., Klein, G., Ersoy, F. and Sanal, Ö., Clin. Exp. Immunol. 35:196-201 (1979).
6. Waldmann, T.A. and Mc Intire, K.R., Lancet 2:1112-1115 (1972).
7. Mc Caw, B.K., Hecht, P., Harnden, D.G. and Teplitz, R.L., Proc. Natl. Acad. Sci. U.S.A. 72:2071-2075 (1975).
8. Cohen, M.M., Sagi, M., Benzur, Z., Schaap, T., Vass R., Kohen, G., Cytogenet. Cell. Genet. 23:44-52 (1979).
9. Gatti, R.A., Bick, M., Tam, C.F., Medici, M.A., Oxelius, V.A., Holland, M., Goldstein, A.L. and Boder, E., Clin. Immunol. Immunopathol (in press).

SOME ASPECTS OF T CELL REGULATION

IN AUTOIMMUNE DISEASES

Rudy E. Ballieux[1,2] and Cobi J. Heijnen[2]

Departments of Clinical Immunology, University Hospital[1]
and University Children's Hospital "Het Wilhelmina
Kinderziekenhuis"[2], Utrecht, The Netherlands

INTRODUCTION

There is ample evidence that the immune response in man is
regulated, although not exclusively, by T cells which have the capacity to induce, amplify or suppress the reactivity of the immune
system. Analogous to the situation in the mouse, these various regulatory T cell functions are exerted by lymphocytes residing in distinct T cell subpopulations (1,2). These subsets can be recognized
by distinct surface markers such as receptors for Fc fragments of
different immunoglobulin isotypes (3) and cell surface structures
defined by monoclonal antibodies (4).

Most studies on the regulatory mechanisms that govern the
humoral immune response in cultures of human peripheral blood
lymphocytes (PBL) have employed systems in which the B cells are
stimulated by polyclonal activators such as Pokeweed mitogen (5,6).
However, experimental conditions have been defined in recent years
which allow for the antigen-specific induction and measurement of
antibody production in vitro by blood lymphocytes (2, 5-8). In our
studies on regulatory T cells in man, we adopted the method for the
generation and quantification of antigen-specific IgM-plaque forming
cells (PFC) as described by Dosch and Gelfand (reviewed in ref. 5).
The present paper deals with the characterization of the various
sets of cells engaged in T cell suppression. In addition it will be
shown that the analysis of an antigen-specific T suppressor (Ts)
cell system in patients with SLE provided essential data for a
better understanding of the T cell interactions in this Ts circuit.

Ts Effector Cells

It has been previously reported (reviewed in ref. 5 and 6) that
the magnitude of the PFC response depends on the concentration of
antigen in the culture. The PFC response drops almost to base line
levels when the cells are cultured with a dose of antigen at least
10-30 times higher than that used to induce optimal plaque formation. This holds both for soluble protein, such as Ovalbumine (OA)
and for cell-bound antigen, such as sheep erythrocytes (SE). It has
been demonstrated earlier by UytdeHaag et al. (9) that the decrease
in PFC response at high dose of antigen is due to activation of
antigen-specific Ts cells which act directly on T helper (Th) cells
and can block helper cell function via soluble antigen-specific
suppressor factors. These Ts effector cells originally have been
localized in the subset of T lymphocytes bearing Fc_γ-receptors
(T_γ^+ cells) (3). Reinherz et al. (10) using monoclonal antibodies
of the OKT series, demonstrated that the T_γ^+ subset is a rather
heterogeneous population of mononuclear cells. In the light of this
observation we attempted to identify the phenotype of the Ts effector cells present in the T_γ^+ subset of human peripheral blood. The
details of this study have been described elsewhere (11), but in
essence the experiment was as follows: purified T_γ^+ cells were
treated with OKT3, OKT4, OKT8 or OKM-1 monoclonal antibodies and
complement. After this treatment the remaining cells were cultured
with supra optimal doses of antigen in order to (re)activate Ts
effector cells. The presence of suppressor effector cell activity
was determined by adding these activated T cell fractions to cultures consisting of Th cells, B cells, adherent cells and an optimum
dose of antigen. The results given in Table 1 show that Ts effector
cells, which are present as such in circulating blood, carry the
phenotype T_γ^+, $T3^+8^+$. No conclusive data are available as yet concerning the presence of the M-1 determinant on antigen-specific Ts
effector cells. Treatment of T_γ^+ cells with OKM-1 and complement

Table 1. Phenotype of the T_γ^+ Suppressor Effector Cell

T_γ^+ Fraction Depleted of Various Subsets	% Suppression After Depletion of Various Subsets
Untreated	$87 \pm 1.9^*$
OKM-1 depleted	71 ± 2.0
OKT3 depleted	16 ± 2.4
OKT4 depleted	73 ± 3.3
OKT8 depleted	-4 ± 0.5

* S.E.M. are given (n=3).

did not influence the suppressor capacity of the remaining cells. This might be due to the fact that the suppression is exerted exclusively by $T_\gamma{}^+3^+8^+M1^-$ cells. However, the possibility still remains that part of the antigen-specific Ts cells are also $M1^+$, as the killing procedures with OKT8 or OKT3 gave also rise to a fall in the percentage of $M1^+T_\gamma{}^+$ cells (11).

Ts Inducer Cells

As reported several years ago (3), the T lymphocyte subset bearing Fcμ-receptors ($T\mu^+$ cells) contains antigen-specific Th cells. However, $T\mu^+$ cells which have been prestimulated with antigen in vitro for 5 or 6 days ('primed' $T\mu^+$ cells) are able to induce Ts effector cell activity in fresh, unprimed T cells (12). This inducing effect of primed $T\mu^+$ cells is antigen-specific (see Heijnen et al. in ref. 2). $T\mu^+$ cells do not exert suppression itself, even after contact with unprimed T cells, but can only activate other T cells to become suppressive (11).

The $T\mu^+$ cell population is heterogeneous when analyzed by monoclonal antibodies. It consists for approximately 70% of $T4^+$ cells and for some 15-20% of $T8^+$ lymphocytes. Antigen-specific Th cells, as defined in a PFC response, are $T4^+$ and consequently carry the phenotype $T\mu^+4^+$. The question was therefore raised as to the nature of the Ts inducer cell within the $T\mu^+$ subset. Would it be different from the $T\mu^+4^+$ helper cell which activates B lymphocytes when stimulated with antigen? In other words: is Th function and Ts inducer function performed by one and the same cell type?

To answer this question, purified $T\mu^+$ cells were treated with either OKT4 or OKT8 and complement. The remaining $T8^+$ depleted $T\mu^+$ cells ($T\mu^+4^+$) and T4 depleted $T\mu^+$ cells ($T\mu^+T8^+$) were tested for Ts inducer activity. As can be seen in Table 2, the addition of

Table 2. Characterization of Human Ts-Inducer Cells

Ts Inducer Cells [*]	Target Culture [*]	PFC/10^6 ly [**]
$-$	5 PBL	1600 ± 24
1 $T\mu^+4^+$	5 PBL	172 ± 7
1 $T\mu^+8^+$	5 PBL	1575 ± 17
0.7 $T\mu^+4^+$ + 0.3 $T\mu^+8^+$	5 PBL	100 ± 8

[*] Cell numbers x 10^6
[**] S.E.M. are given (n=3).

primed $T\mu^{+}8^{+}$ lymphocytes to target cultures did not lead to suppression, whereas the addition of antigen-primed $T\mu^{+}4^{+}$ cells resulted in suppression. Thus, Th and Ts inducer cells both carry the phenotype $T\mu^{+}4^{+}$. Also the use of the monoclonal antibody 5/9, which in the PWM system defines a small subset of T cells within the $T4^{+}$ population containing all Th activity (13), did not allow for distinction between Th and Ts inducer cells. On the other hand, it could be shown that Th and Ts inducer cells can be distinguished by a different sensitivity of their respective $Fc\mu R$ to treatment with theophylline (Heijnen et al. in ref. 2), by certain allo anti-sera (14) and by antibodies present in the serum of certain patients with juvenile rheumatoid arthritis (15). A further clearcut difference between these two functional subsets is the fact that Ts-inducer cells can be stimulated directly by antigen, whereas for the activation of Th cells the presence of HLA-D identical monocytes is required (Heijnen et al. in ref. 2).

Ts Precursor Cells

Once the information was obtained that Ts inducer cells form a distinct subset of $T\mu^{+}T4^{+}$ cells, experiments were designed to characterize the target cells for the primed Ts inducer cell. To that end primed $T\mu^{+}$ cells were added to cultures containing B cells and T cells of subsets characterized by different phenotypes and stimulated with an optimal dose of antigen. It can be concluded from the data in Table 3 that the interaction of primed $T\mu^{+}$ inducer cells with T lymphocytes, lacking receptors for the Fc fragments of IgG and IgM leads to suppression. It has been shown by Palacios et al. (16) that the $T_{\mu\gamma}^{-}$ subset almost completely overlaps with the subset of T cells which form rosettes with autologous erythro-

Table 3. Characterization of the Target T Cells for
          Primed Ts Inducer Cells

Ts Inducer (Primed $T\mu^{+}$ cells)[*]	T Cells Added to the Assay System[*][†]	PFC/10^{6} ly
1.0	0.5 T[**]	364
1.0	0.5 $T\mu^{+}$	3414
1.0	0.5 T_{γ}^{+}	2167
1.0	0.5 $T_{\mu\gamma}^{-}$	283

[*] Cell number x 10^{6}
[†] Assay system: 1.5 B cells, 2.0 T cells and 5 SE.
[**] Unprimed, unselected, autologous T cells

cytes (Tar$^+$). The Tar$^+$ subset is considered to represent the post-thymic precursor T cell population. The data in Table 3 indicate therefore that primed Tμ^+ cells can induce Tar$^+$ cells to become Ts effector cells. Because the T$_{\mu\gamma}^-$ or Tar$^+$ subset is a rather hetero-geneous pool of T cells (17), we tried to characterize the target for the Ts inducer cell in more detail. To that end unprimed T cells were fractionated into Tar$^+$ and Tar$^-$ cell populations. The Tar$^+$ cells were divided into 3 portions and treated with the monoclonal anti-bodies OKT4, OKT8 or medium. After incubation with complement, the re-maining cells were tested for the presence of Ts precursor cells in cultures stimulated with primed T$_\mu^+$ suppressor inducer cells.

The results summarized in Table 4 indicate that only the T8$^+$ subset of Tar$^+$ population contains Ts precursor cells. However, optimum suppression was achieved only in cultures of T8$^+$ar$^+$ lympho-cytes if T4$^+$ ar$^+$ cells were also present. Therefore the target for the Ts inducer cell is a T8$_{\mu\gamma}^-$ar$^+$ lymphocyte.

Defects in Ts Circuit in SLE Patients

The interesting question now came up: does the T8$^+_{\mu\gamma}^-$ar$^+$ pre-cursor cell differentiate _in vitro_ to a T8$^+\gamma^+$ ar$^-$ Ts effector cell which is identical to the earlier defined T$_\gamma^+$ effector cell present _in vivo_ in peripheral blood and lymphoid organs? On the basis of detailed analysis of the phenotypes the answer is: yes. Support for this conclusion came from the analysis of the defect in the suppres-sor T cell circuit in patiens with SLE.

Table 4.   Phenotype of Ts Precursor Cells in the Tar$^+$ Subset

Ts Inducer (Primed T$_\mu^+$ cells)	T Cells Added to the Assay System*†	% of Control PFC Response
0.5	–	100
0.5	1.0 Tar$^+$	18
0.5	2.0 Tar$^+$	21
0.5	1.0 T4$^+$ar$^+$	80
0.5	2.0 T4$^+$ar$^+$	97
0.5	1.0 T8$^+$ar$^+$	43
0.5	2.0 T8$^+$ar$^+$	38
0.5	0.5 T4$^+$ar$^+$ + 0.5 T8$^+$ar$^+$	17

[*] Cell numbers x 10^6
[†] Assay system: 1.5 B cells, 2.0 Tar$^+$ - depleted T cells and 3 μg OA/ml.

It has previously been reported by a great number of investigators that ConA induced suppressor T cell activity can be disturbed
in patients with SLE. In addition it was shown by Gladman et al. (18)
and by our group (19) that also antigen-specific Ts activity in
these patiens is defective. This has been documented particularly
for the high antigen dose activation of Ts effector cells, which we
discussed earlier. However, Heijnen et al. (19) has recently reported
that also the 'feedback suppressor T cell circuit' in SLE patients
can be disturbed. In a number of patients in an active stages of the
disease a co-culture of primed Ts inducer cells and Ts precursor
cells did not result in the generation of Ts effector cells. By
recombination experiments it could be shown that Ts inducer cells
of these patients could function normally. However, the defect in
this suppressor circuit in SLE patients is based on the functional
absence of Ts precursor cells (11,19). This finding is in agreement
with the reported absence of Tar^+ cells in PBL of SLE patients in
the active stage of the disease. It could be established that the
absence of $T\gamma^+8^+ar^-$ effector suppressor cells in these patients
always coincides with the absence of $T_{\mu\gamma}^-8^+ar^+$ suppressor precursor
cells (19). These findings in patients with SLE as well as the data
on the phenotypic and functional similarities between the in vitro
generated and the in vivo present T suppressor effector cells suggest that these cells are identical and thus derived from the same
precursor cell. Hence, the Ts circuit depicted in Fig. 1, which
reflects the results of experiments in vitro, may be operative in
man in vivo as well.

ACKNOWLEDGMENTS

    This study was supported in part by the Foundation for Medical
Research (FUNGO; grantnumber 13-40-91), which is subsidized by the

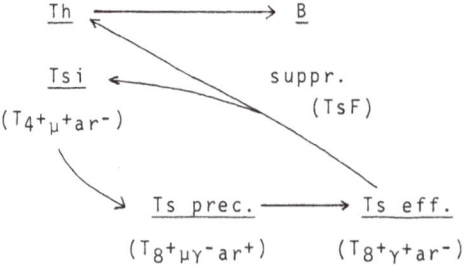

Fig. 1.   Ts circuit in man. Th = T helper cell; Tsi = suppressor
          inducer cell; Ts prec = T suppressor precursor cell;
          Ts eff. = T suppressor effector cell which acts on Tsi
          and Th via a soluble T cell suppressor factor TsF.

Netherlands Organisation for the Advancement of Pure Research
(Z.W.O.).

REFERENCES

1. Gershon, R.K., J. Allergy Clin. Immunol. 66:18 (1980).
2. Fauci, A.S., Ballieux, R.E. (eds.), "Human B cell function:
   activation and immunoregulation," Raven Press, New York (1982).
3. Heijnen, C.J., UytdeHaag, F., Gmelig-Meyling, F.H.J., Ballieux,
   R.E., Cell. Immunol. 43:282 (1979).
4. Reinherz, E.L., Schlossman, S.F., Immunol. Today 2:69 (1981).
5. Fauci, A.S., Ballieux, R.E. (eds.), "Antibody production in man:
   in vitro synthesis and clinical implications," Academic Press,
   New York (1979).
6. Möller, G., Immunol. Rev. 45:3 (1979).
7. Lane, H.C., Volkman, D.J., Whalen, G., Fauci, A.S., J. Exp. Med.
   154:1043 (1981).
8. Misiti, J., Waldmann, T.A., J. Exp. Med. 154:1069 (1981).
9. UytdeHaag, F., Heijnen, C.J., Pot, K.H., Ballieux, R.E.,
   J. Immunol. 126:503 (1981).
10. Reinherz, E.L., Moretta, L., Roper, M., Breard, J.M., Mingari,
    M.C., Cooper, M.D., Schlossman, S.F., J. Exp. Med. 151:969
    (1980).
11. Heijnen, C.J., Pot, K.H., Ballieux, R.E., Eur. J. Immunol..
    (in press).
12. Heijnen, C.J., UytdeHaag, F., Pot, C.H., Ballieux, R.E., Nature
    280:589 (1979).
13. Corte G, Mingari, M.C., Moretta, A., Damiani, G., Moretta, L.,
    Bargellesi, A., J. Immunol. 128:16 (1982).
14. Leeuwen, A. van, Festenstein, H., Rood, J. J. van, J. Exp. Med.
    152:235s (1980).
15. Reinherz, E.L., Strelkauskas, A.J., O'Brien, C., Schlossman
    S.F., J. Immunol. 123:83 (1980).
16. Palacios, R., Alarcon-Segovia, D., Llorente, L., Ruiz-Arguelles,
    A., Diaz-Jouanen, E., Immunology 42:127 (1981).
17. Heijnen, C.J., UytdeHaag, F., Ballieux, R.E., Immunopathol.
    3:63 (1980).
18. Gladman, D., Keystone, E., Urowitz, M., Cane, D., Poplonski,
    L., Clin. Exp. Immunol. 40:77 (1980).
19. Heijnen, C.J., Pot, K.H., Kater, L., Kluin-Nelemans, H.C.,
    UytdeHaag, F., Ballieux, R.E., Clin. Exp. Immunol. 47:359
    (1982).

EARLY DETECTION OF AUTOIMMUNE ENDOCRINE DISORDERS

Deborah Doniach and Gian Franco Bottazzo

The Department of Immunology
Middlesex Hospital Medical School
London W1, UK

INTRODUCTION

Organ specific autoimmunity (AI) has been demonstrated in all
the defined endocrine organs except the pineal gland and is now
being studied in the paracrine systems of the gastrointestinal tract
and the hypothalamus. The 'autoimmune' endocrine disorders are characterized by the presence of antibodies in the patients' serum
which may be detected years before the onset of clinical symptoms
and are useful monitors of the lesions well before hormonal deficiencies can be measured by metabolic tests. In the case of
'stimulating' antibodies that produce hormone excess, and hormone
receptor antibodies generally, the situation is far more complex.

In this review we will describe the present range of tissue
antibodies helpful in early diagnosis and try to show that substantial morbidity could be avoided by preventive autoimmune screening
in selected individuals.

WHO ARE THE SUSCEPTIBLE INDIVIDUALS?

Screening for tissue antibodies has been carried out on a population basis in several countries (1,2) and showed a similar
distribution of autoantibodies in most continents except Africa
where autoimmunity is rare due to the overriding 'take-over'
effects of parasitic infections upon the resources of the immune
system.

The AI endocrine diseases all have a strong genetic element.
For instance in Graves' thyrotoxicosis, in Hashimoto's disease and
in juvenile onset diabetes, the concordance rate of the clinical
conditions is about 50% in monozygotic twins. This contrasts strik-
ingly with the non-organ-specific collagen disorders such as SLE and
rheumatoid arthritis, where only 10% of identical twins are both
affected. The frequency of the endocrine immunopathies varies tre-
mendously from common conditions such as the thyroid autoimmune
diseases and AI gastritis through to insulin dependent diabetes, AI
adrenalitis and gonadal atrophy to the rare autoimmune hypophysitis
and parathyroid atrophies. The more common the disease, the greater
the frequency of antibodies to that particular organ in the population, and more so in close relatives of the affected patient. In
addition, many of these diseases have a predilection for the female
sex and tend to be expressed in adult life, so that antibodies are
most likely to be found in middleaged women especially those belong-
ing to 'autoimmune families'. To a certain extent, the prevalence
and titres of autoantibodies also go with the size of the endocrine
organs, presumably in relation to the total amount of antigenic
material made available to the regulating networks of autoreactive
immunocytes.

A most important feature in this group of disorders is the
striking overlap between them. At the extreme end we have the rare
'polyendocrine' syndromes where all the endocrine organs may be
involved in the same patient. These cases have been recognized clinically for over 60 years and have received growing attention since
the discovery of islet-cell antibodies in insulin dependent diabetes
(IDDM) and the identification of pituitary autoimmunity (3,4).

The classical polyendocrine syndromes include Schmidt's syndrome
(thyroiditis and adrenalitis with or without IDDM) and the candida-
endocrinopathy or C-E syndrome mostly seen in pediatric practice (5).
There are also far more complex mixtures. Endocrine autoimmunity may
be associated with diseases such as chronic active hepatitis or
myasthenia gravis; with AI haemolytic anaemia or thrombocytopenia
and with malabsorption syndromes. In these cases the immune defects
are of a wider scope and include immunoglobulin deficiencies, commonly of the IgA class, severe allergies and various thymus
dependent-(T)-lymphocyte defects. These abnormalities can be identified in various members of the family as well as in the patients
themselves (6).

Much more common are the 'thyrogastric' syndromes, i.e. a combination of thyroid and gastric autoimmunity. Usually the patient
presents clinically with one or other of these common conditions
i.e. a thyroid disease or pernicious anemia. Their serum often
contains a number of relevant and interesting mixtures of organ-
specific antibodies, some of which are indicative of a subclinical
lesion that can be followed and prevented from becoming troublesome

or dangerous to the patients's well being. It is in this category
of 'serological polyendocrinopathy' that our best chances of preventive measures will gradually emerge in coming years. The diffi-
culty today is that for most of the organs except thyroid, it is not
known what proportion of patients with circulating antibodies eventually express the corresponding clinical disorder. There is an
urgent need to test predisposed subjects for all available specific-
ities in relation to the endocrine system. At the same time it is
advisable to look for the non-organ-specific markers as the overlap
which extends towards the other end of the autoimmune spectrum is
not well understood.

We can now define the susceptible groups:

1. Patients with recognized autoimmunity to one organ.

2. Their first degree relatives, especially sibs and offspring
of both sexes.

3. Patients with non-endocrine disorders known to overlap or
be connected with the AI endocrinopathies (for instance PA, RA,
coeliac/malabsorption syndromes, AI liver diseases, vitiligo and
alopecia).

4. The relatives of group (3).

5. Detailed family histories are most important in relation to
autoimmunity and any patient with a positive FH should be screened.

6. Patients with disorders of unknown aetiology. The presence
of autoantibodies may give a clue for new interpretations or fresh
discoveries (e.g. hypothalamic antibodies in diabetes insipidus).

7. Middle-aged women generally, especially those presenting in
outpatient departments with fatigue, depression or other ill-
defined symptoms.

DETECTION OF ORGAN ANTIBODIES

The range of autoantibodies that can be detected for the early
diagnosis of endocrine diseases are shown in Tables 1 and 2. The
most suitable method is still the indirect immunofluorescence test
(IFT) done on unfixed cryostat sections of human organs obtained
at operations, or soon after death, from renal transplant donors.
For anterior pituitary, ovarian and hypothalamic antibodies fresh
baboon glands or brain tissue have proved easier to obtain and
convenient to handle. The crossreactivity of human antibodies with
primate organs is high compared with guinea-pig, rat or mouse
tissues, which cannot be used for this type of work. Fixatives are

Table 1. Diagnostic Antibodies for Endocrine Autoimmune Disorders

Disease	Antibodies[†] react with	Frequency in normal population
Graves' thyrotoxicosis	TSH receptors (Table 2)	nyd
Some nontoxic nodular sporadic goitres	Thyroid microsomes (HA)	F>M; 0–20% according to sex and age
Primary myxoedema	Thyroglobulin (HA)	F>M; 0–20% according to sex and age
Endocrine exophthalmos	Extraocular muscle (ELISA) retroorbital tissues	nyd
Pernicious anaemia	Intrinsic factor (RIA)	0.1%
	Gastric parietal cell	F>M; 0–16% according to sex and age
Fundal (type A) gastritis	Gastric parietal cell	F>M; 0–16% according to sex and age
Antral (type B) gastritis	Gastrin cell	0.1%
Addison's disease	Adrenal cortex	0.1%
Premature menopause with adrenalitis	Adrenal cortex	0.1%
Primary gonadal deficiency	Steroid cells, gonadal and placental	0.01%
	Sperm and ovum	
Idiopathic hypoparathyroidism	? parathyroid chief cells	7%
Insulin-dependent diabetes	Pancreatic islet cells;	nyd
	1. 'Common antigen'	0.5%
	2. Insulin cell	nyd
	3. Glucagon cell	0.2%
	4. Somatostatin cell	0.5%
	5. Anterior pituitary cells	nyd

Partial pituitary deficiency	Prolactin cell	0.1%
	Growth hormone cell	0.01%
Idiopathic central diabetes insipidus	Hypothalamic vasopressin and/or oxytocin cells	0.01%
Vitiligo	Melanocyte	nyd
Myasthenia gravis	Acetylcholine receptors (RIA)	1%
Autoimmune liver disorders (overlap with endocrine AI)		
Chronic active liver disease		
Lupoid variant	Nuclei (mostly diffuse)	F>M; 0–20% according to sex and age
	Smooth muscle (mostly actin)	12%
Liver and kidney microsome variant	Liver and kidney microsome	0.3%
Cholestatic variant	Mitochondria	0.4–0.7%
Primary biliary cirrhosis	Mitochondrial inner membranes	0.4–0.7%

† Detected by immunofluorescence unless otherwise stated.
nyd = not yet determined
HA = Haemagglutination with antigen coated red cells.
RIA = Radioimmunoassay
ELISA = enzyme-linked-immunosorbant assay

not recommended as they often inactivate the cellular autoantigens. The test can be done on several organs at once and requires only a few drops of serum from the patient. Semiquantitative tests are obtained by repeating positive results of undiluted serum on suitable dilutions to endpoint. The old-established tests with thyroid, stomach or adrenal and more recently pancreatic islets are available in many laboratories but for the more recent endocrine cell antibodies such as pituitary, gonadal and hypothalamic, the tests are at present only done in specialized research units. These organs should be easier to obtain in future, since an American firm (Biodex, New Jersey) sends monkey organ sections ready processed to any country on request at a reasonable cost. For thyroglobulin and thyroid microsomal antibodies, immunofluorescence has been superceded by passive haemagglutination (HA) performed with commercial kits of sheep or turkey red cells coated with the purified human antigens (Welcome Reagents, London, and Fujizoki, Tokyo). The older complement fixation tests have been abandoned in favour of immunofluorescence done with anticomplement (C3) serum conjugated with fluorescein (green) or rhodamine (red). It is now clear that only a proportion of any organ antibodies fix complement and that this subset is more pertinent to the pathogenesis of autoimmune lesions such as pancreatic insulitis in diabetes. This probably applies equally to other endocrinopathies so that the standard IFT with anti-immunoglobulin conjugates should be combined with the complement fixing immunofluorescent test (ICFT) for predictive studies. Radiometric assays become possible when purified antigens are available. Receptor antibody tests will be discussed separately. A method which will be of great value in future is the enzyme linked immunosorbant assay (ELISA). This is at present being used to detect ocular muscle antibodies as a test for endocrine exophthalmos (7). The 'monoclonal antibody revolution' is being applied in this work and in the analysis of hormone receptor structure (6). Monoclonal antibodies are a useful tool for the purification and separation of endocrine autoantigens.

EARLY DETECTION IN SPECIFIC DISEASES

Adrenalitis

There are clinical circumstances where autoantibody tests done at an early stage can actually be life-saving. These are the cases of subclinical adrenal deficiency who develop an adrenal crisis during infection or acute appendicitis. There are descriptions in the literature of young patients with unsuspected Addison's disease who come in as emergencies and die before a diagnosis can be reached. Some of these are known to have had thyroid disease in the past or they suffer from insulin-dependent diabetes. Some have secondary amenorrhoea associated with steroid cell gonadal antibodies. Others have an undiagnosed hypophysitis. Screening for adrenal and

pituitary antibodies would be of particular benefit in these circumstances.

Infertility and Amenorrhoea

A proportion of patients with no clinical signs of anterior
pituitary failure except for absence of periods and inability to
become pregnant, were found to have antibodies to prolaction cells.
The percentage of positive sera appears to depend mainly on the selection of cases and varied between 5% and 30%. Further studies are
urgently needed in this interesting field. For instance it is not
yet known if any of the patients with microadenomas of the prolactin
cells ever have autoantibodies. Cases are now appearing in the literature where a prolactinoma is diagnosed but where pituitary histo-
logy showed enlargment of the anterior lobe with lymphocytic hypophysitis, reminiscent of the appearances in the thyroid gland in
Hashimoto goitres (8).

Some girls with primary or secondary amenorrhoea have no indication of adrenal failure, yet their sera contain adrenal antibodies
and steroid cell antibodies reacting with Leydig cells in the testis
and ovarian steroid cells. It is not known how many such cases will
eventually develop clinical Addison's disease. Early detection and
careful follow up of these young people will teach us a great deal
about polyendocrine autoimmunity in its milder forms.

Pancreatic Insulitis

Patients with autoimmune thyroiditis, gastritis or adrenalitis
have an increased risk of developing insulin dependent diabetes at
any age. Islet cell antibodies of the complement fixing variety
(CF-ICA) are more closely associated with the presence of an active
insulitis because among the mixture of different serum antibodies,
some CF-ICA are directed specifically to the pancreatic beta-cells
that secrete insulin. Only the beta-cells are destroyed in diabetes,
and it is this specific subset which is cytotoxic and relevant. At
present it looks as though about half of the subjects with CF-ICA
in their sera develop diabetes. This is based upon a 4-year follow-
up of 'unaffected' first degree relatives of diabetic children and
a 6 year observation of 'endocrine' patients who happened to have
a positive CF-ICA when screened for various tissue reactions (9).

It is regretable that we do not yet know how to reverse an
ongoing insulitis. However, it is obvious that before a suitable
form of treatment can be discovered it is necessary to know exactly
who is liable to develop diabetes in future years, Extensive glucose
tolerance testing in past research schemes has not led to reliable
predictions because the tests remain normal until some 80-90% of

the beta-cells are lost, much as in the case of atrophic thyroiditis.

The recent finding that cyclosporin-A can prevent diabetes in
the BB rat model makes it likely that the drug will be tried in diabetic families. The BB rat develops insulitis and thyroiditis and
has a strong resemblance to the human disease (10).

Atrophic Thyroiditis

Myxoedema often comes on so insiduously that it is easy to miss
it unless one is constantly on the look out for early signs. Routine
screening of middleaged women shows a 20% prevalence of thyroid antibodies but only 10-20% of the positive reactors eventually lose
some of their thyroid function. Because of the much greater frequency of thyroiditis compared with insulitis or adrenalitis, even this
low figure represents a substantial number of patients. The TRH/TSH
test offers the best chance of selecting hypothyroid cases prospec-
tively, because antibody tests by themselves do not distinguish
between the progressive form of thyroiditis and the harmless focal
variety. In our clinic we give thyroxine replacement to any patients
with a raised basal serum TSH (i.e. higher than 6 mU/1). When this
is normal but the value rises above 30 mU at 20 minutes after 200 ug
TRH/iv, then we give a trial of T4 for 6 months and see if the TRH
returns to normal 3 months after stopping the replacement.

It is still hoped that future studies with thyroid-growth-
blocking antibodies will help us to select the progressive cases
more accurately but we need an easier method than the cytochemical
bio-assays used so far (11).

Autoimmune Gastritis

Atrophic fundal gastritis is known to exist in one third of
all patients with autoimmune thyroiditis but as in the case of
thyroid atrophy, many remain totally subclinical during the whole
of the patient's life and neither the presence of parietal cell antibodies nor their titre are reliable indices of progression.
Pernicious anaemia occurs 5-8 times more frequently than expected
in patients with thyroid disease and the easiest way to monitor this
possibility is by measuring the serum B_{12} level at intervals. The
radioimmunoassay with labeled vitamin B_{12} for intrinsic factor antibodies should also be carried out as it is positive in over half
the cases of latent pernicious anaemia. The presence of these antibodies in the gastric juice would probably be more reliable for
prediction but since the antibodies are combined with intrinsic
factor it is difficult to extract them from the immune complexes
and symptomless patients are not willing to have gastric intuba-
tions.

Table 2. Recognized 'Receptor Antibody Diseases'

Disease	Receptor reacting with antibodies	Action of antibodies
Graves thyrotoxicosis	TSH-R (TSI)	Stimulation of T3/T4 synthesis
Graves' with goitre	? TSH-R (TGI)	Stimulation of cell division
Sporadic/familial non toxic nodular goitre	? TSH-R (TGI)	Stimulation of cell division
Primary myxoedema	TSH-R (TSI-block) (TGI-block)	Blocking of c-AMP stimulation Blocking of cell division
Atrophic fundal gastritis	Gastrin-R on parietal cells	Blocking of carbonic anhydrase ? blocking of parietal cell regeneration
Myasthenia gravis	Acetylcholine-R	Blocking of neuromuscular transmission
Bronchial Asthma	Beta-adrenergic-R	Impaired sensitivity to beta-adrenergic drugs
Insulin resistent diabetes	Insulin-R	Blocking of insulin secretion Insulin-like action on adipocytes
Oestrogen-resistant gonadal deficiency	Oestrogen-R on ovarian cells	Blocking of oestrogen responses ? blocking of steroid cell regeneration
Renal failure	Parathormone-R	Blocking of parathyroid hormone action on target organs

Atrophic gastritis can contribute to iron deficiency anaemia by blood leakage from the injured gastric mucosa, and parietal cell antibodies are often found in women presenting with this common condition.

AUTOIMMUNITY TO HORMONE-AND OTHER CELL RECEPTORS

The best known autoimmune 'receptor' disease is Graves' thyrotoxicosis. TSH-receptor antibodies have been demonstrated in the serum of these patients for over 25 years by numerous methods (Table 2) and are thought to cause the hypersecretion of triiodothyronine and thyroxine (T3/T4). As a generic term 'thyroid stimulating antibodies' or TSAb is suitable but the autoimmunity is always polyclonal and each patient responds differently to a range of epitopes or antigenic sites on the complex structure of the hormone receptor so that some antibodies 'bind' to it, some transmit a message to synthesise hormones, some give signals for cell division and goitre formation and some block the receptors and prevent them from responding to TSH or to other TSAb (12). Many of these antibodies can coexist in a single patient or come and go at different times of life. This is the reason for the great variety of clinical signs and symptoms seen in Graves' disease and in other autoimmune 'receptor' disorders (13). It is likely that endocrine exophthalmos is a separate autoimmunization to eye components but the fact that 90% of cases are somehow related to past, present or future thyroid dysfunction, suggests that there is an immunological relationship. It is of special interest that one of the monoclonal antibodies produced by a mouse hybridoma after immunization with eye muscle antigens cross-reacted with the principal antigen of human thyroiditis, i.e. the microsomal antigen (7). Another hybridoma made with lymphocytes from a patient with pretibial myxoedema has the property of stimulating fibroblast growth (14). To add further complexity these antibodies cross-react with different affinities with the TSH receptors of other animal species that are used for detecting TSAb.

New simplified assays for the early diagnosis of thyrotoxicosis are being developed using a continuous line of rat thyroid cells immortalized with intact function. There is hope of combining c-AMP stimulation and radioiodine uptake with thymidine incorporation in the same cultures. This will measure both hormone stimulating and growth stimulating antibodies in a reproducible manner. Thyroid growth-stimulating antibodies are detected in some sporadic non toxic nodular goitres (11) and this may represent a new form of thyroid autoimmunity despite the usual absence in this disease of conventional thyroglobulin or thyroid microsomal antibodies in the serum, or lymphocytic thyroid gland infiltrates (15). When the tests become easier to perform they will prove of help in deciding whether or not to operate on any given patient and how much of the

gland to remove as high titres of the 'Growth-antibodies' (TGI) are
associated with postoperative recurrences in nontoxic nodular
goitres (16). Also, if TGI are present it is probably ineffective
to treat the patient with thyroxine replacement as pituitary TSH is
suppressed by the receptor antibodies.

Other receptor antibodies have been identified and are used for
early diagnosis. An important radioimmunoassay using radioactive
bungarotoxin is regularly used for the early diagnosis of myasthenia
gravis. The test is quite sensitive and very specific. Another pub-
licized receptor disease is the rare insulin resistant diabetes with
acanthosis nigricans, where insulin receptor antibodies can be
detected on the patient's circulating monocytes and in the serum
with labelled insulin in a radioreceptor assay. At present only the
most severe form of this disease is recognized but already there
are reports of cases where hypoglycaemia was the presenting feature
rather than insulin resistance and it can be anticipated that more
chronic cases will be found. Nearly all the patients with insulin-
receptor antibodies have ribonucleoprotein precipitating antibodies
and 'speckled' anti-nuclear antibody patterns in the immunofluorescence tests for ANA. Many of the cases have evidence of Sjogren's
sicca syndrome. Other less well characterized receptor antibodies
are those found in some cases of asthma which are directed to the
beta-adrenergic receptors and antibodies to the parathormone receptors found in chronic renal failure. In relation to endocrine
disorders (17) it is of interest that antibodies to the oestrogen
receptors on ovarian cells account for some cases of ovarian atrophy
in patients with coexisting myasthenia gravis giving rise to
oestrogen resistant hypogonadism.

Full discussion of these autoimmune 'receptor' diseases are
found in the recent Ciba Symposium on "Receptors, Antibodies and
Disease"(13). Radioreceptor tests are available commercially for
TSAb but most of the other methods are still in the research stage
and are difficult to apply in clinical practice.

FUTURE PROSPECTS

Autoimmunity to the anterior pituitary and hypothalamus and
antibodies directed to endocrine cells of the gut such as CIP-and
secretin-cells, are at present being studied and their significance
for early diagnosis is being worked out. One of the remarkable
findings is that in diabetic families, some relatives who had islet-
cell antibodies without being diabetic, reacted with several of the
anterior pituitary cells (multicell pattern) (18).

These antibodies were still present in newly diagnosed IDDM
but disappeared with time. This could indicate that pituitary autoimmunity of a distinct kind from the known lymphocytic hypophysitis,

could play a role in the initiation of the pathogenic events that
eventually lead to breakdown of glucose homeostasis in some forms
of diabetes. Gut endocrine cells also appear involved in diabetes
mellitus and in coeliac disease and other malabsorption syndromes
(19). Exploration of the hypothalamus with its numerous endocrine
cells has only recently been undertaken due to the known clinical
association of central idiopathic diabetes insipidus with other
autoimmune disorders. Nearly 40% of such cases proved to have cytoplasmic autoantibodies that could be detected by IFT on section of
the supraoptic nuclei and paraventricular nuclei. This could be of
diagnostic help in distinguishing the 'functional' and 'secondary'
case of diabetes insipidus from those due to destruction of vaso-
pressin cells in the hypothalamus (20).

The future will reveal many more autoimmune reactions connected
with receptors to hormones and neurotransmitters. With the help of
monoclonal antibodies it will be possible to purify specific receptors and develop sensitive radiometric or other technologically
advanced methods that will make it possible to diagnose early stages
of endocrine diseases.

The DR region of the major histocompatibility HLA complex is
involved in regulating lymphocyte networks and the endocrine immunopathies are more prevalent in subjects with DR3, DR4 and DR5. HLA
typing helps to predict recurrences in thyrotoxicosis (21) and has
been used to select susceptible relatives in diabetic families (22).

REFERENCES

1. Hooper, B., Whittingham, S., Mathews, J.D., Mackay, I.R.,
    Curnow, D.H., Clin. Exp. Immunol. 12:79-87 (1972).
2. Tunbridge, W.M.G., Brewis, M., French, J.M., Br. Med. J.   ·
    282:258-262 (1982).
3. Battazzo, G.F., Florin-Christensen, A., Doniach, D., Lancet
    2:1279-1283 (1974).
4. Battazzo, G.F., Pouplard, D., Florin-Christensen, A., Doniach,
    D., Lancet 2:97-101 (1975).
5. Neufeld, M., MacLaren, N., Blizzard, R.M., Pediatr. Ann.
    9:43-53 (1980).
6. Fellows, R.E., Eisenbarth, G.S. (eds.), in: "Monoclonal Anti-
    bodies in Endocrine Research", Raven Press, New York (1981).
7. Kodoma, K., Sikorska, H., Bandy-Dafoe, P., Bayly, R., Wall,
    J.R., Lancet 2:1353-1356 (1982).
8. Doniach, D., Cudworth, A.G., Khoury, E.L., Battazzo, G.F.,
    in: "Recent Progress in Endocrinology", O'Riordan, J.L.H. (ed.),
    Churchill, Livingstone, Edinburgh, 2:99-131 (1982).
9. Battazzo, G.F., Mirakian, R., Dean, B.M., McNally, J.M.,
    Doniach, D., in: "The Genetics of Diabetes", Tattersall, R.B.,
    Koberling, J. (eds.), 1982 Serono Symposium, 47:79-90.

10. Laupacis, A., Stiller, C.R., Gardell, C., Keown, P., Dupre, J., Wallace, A.C., Thibert, P., Lancet 1:10-12 (1983).
11. Drexhage, H.A., Chayen, J., Bitensky, L., Battazzo, G.F., Doniach, D., in: "Cytochemical Bioassay Techniques and Applications", Chayen, J., Bitensky, L. (eds.), Dekker, New York (1983) (in press).
12. Battazzo, G.F., Drexhage, H.A., Khoury, E.L. in: "Receptors, Antibodies and Disease", Evered, D., Whelan, J. (eds.), Ciba Foundation Symposium 90, Pitman, London (1980).
13. "Receptors, Antibodies and Disease", Pitman, London, CIBA Symposium 90 (1982).
14. Kohn, L.D., Personal Communication, 1982.
15. Doniach, D., Chiovato, L., Hanafusa, T., Battazzo, G.F., in: "Seminar in Immunopathology: Immunopathology of Cell Surface Receptors", Mackay, J., Miescher, P.A. (eds.), Berlin Springer Seminars in Immunopathology (1982) (in press).
16. Chiovato, L., Hammond, L.J., Hanfusa, T., Pujol-Borrell, R., Doniach, D., Battazzo, G.F., Clin. Endocrinol. (1983) (in press).
17. Volpe, R., Autoimmunity in the Endocrine System", Berlin Springer Monographs on Endocrionology (1981).
18. Mirakian, R., Cudworth, A.G., Battazzo, G.F., Richardson, C.A., Doniach, D., Lancet 2:755-760 (1982).
19. Mirakian, R., Richardson, C.A., Battazzo, G.F., Doniach, D., Clin. Immunol. Newsletter 2:161-167 (1981).
20. Scherbaum, V.A., Battazzo, G.F., Lancet (1983) (in press).
21. Farid, N.R. (ed.) "HLA in Endocrine and Metabolic Disorders", New York, Academic Press (1981).
22. Doniach, D., Battazzo, G.F., Drexhage, H.A., in: "Clinical Aspects of Immunology", 2:903, Lachmann, P.J., Peters, K. (eds.), Oxford Blackwell (1982).

PERMANENT LINES OF T LYMPHOCYTES SPECIFIC FOR ACETYLCHOLINE RECEPTORS: A CLONAL APPROACH TO STUDY THE PATHOGENESIS OF MYASTHENIA GRAVIS

B.C.G. Schalke, R. Hohlfeld[+], I. Kalies[*], A. Ben-Nun[o,**],
I.R. Cohen[o] and H. Wekerle

Clinical Research Unit for Multiple Sclerosis
Max-Planck-Society, D-8700 Würzburg, F.R.G.
Department of Cell Biology, Weizmann Institute[o]
Rehovot, Israel

INTRODUCTION

Myasthenia gravis is a disease of the neuromuscular synapse. Studies during the past decade have unequivocally established that the pathogenic defect in myasthenia is due to autoantibodies specific for the nicotinic acetylcholine receptors (AChR) of the end plate. These autoantibodies were demonstrated to bind to receptor bearing areas (1), they can transfer disease to formerly normal recipient animals (2), and cause accelerated receptor decay on the postsynaptic membranes (3). Humoral antibodies reflect, however, only one aspect of the autoimmune pathogenesis of myasthenia gravis. 1) There is strong evidence that, in addition, autoimmune T lymphocytes are critically involved in the pathogenesis of myasthenia gravis. This is most probably true in the afferent stages of the disease mechanism, and possibly also in the effector phase. The evidence for T cell participation in myasthenia gravis seems to be (loosely) linked to certain determinants of the human major histocompatibility gene complex, HLA (4). It is known that the immune response genes coded for within the major histocompatibility complex predominantly act in T cell dependent stages of the immune response (5). 2) Some, but possibly not all patients with myasthenia gravis possess peripheral

Present addresses:
[+] Neurological University Hospital, Düsseldorf, F.R.G.
[*] Institute of Clinical Immunology, University, Erlangen, F.R.G.
[**] Sidney Farber Cancer Center, Harvard University, Boston, MA, USA.

blood lymphocytes reactive against isolated acetylcholine receptors
by proliferation (6) or by secretion of lymphokines (7). 3) Most,
if not all pathogenic anti-acetylcholine receptor autoantibodies
belong to the IgG isotype (8). IgG synthesis depends on interaction
between helper T lymphocytes with antibody secreting B lymphocytes (9). 4) In most cases of myasthenia gravis, the thymus is pathologically changed. Evidence is accumulating that in fact the thymus
is the primary focus of the disease. Since the thymus is the central
site of T cell formation, it appears plausible that thymic T lymphocytes are in first line involved in the intrathymic phase of myasthenia gravis (10).

    The most direct approach to study the role of autoimmune T lym-
phocytes in the pathogenesis of myasthenia gravis is to isolate such
cells from a myasthenic immune system, to purify and propagate the
relevant T lymphocytes in vitro, and to study their functional capacities either in vivo or in vitro. Our laboratory has been involved
in demonstration and analyses of autoreactive T lymphocytes for
several years. In the case of Experimental Autoimmune Orchitis we
developed a system which allowed the isolation of testis specific
autoimmune T lymphocytes in vitro (11). These T cells were able to
transfer disease, when reapplied to compatible recipient animals (12). We adapted this approach to study AChR-specific T cells
in the pathogenesis of Experimental Autoimmune Myasthenia Gravis
(EAMG).

Purification of pluriclonal T lymphocyte populations specific for AChR

    AChR-specific T lymphocyte populations were isolated following
a combined in vivo/in vitro selection procedure (13). We immunized
inbred Lewis rats according to a schedule, which reliably leads to
induction of EAMG. About 9-14 days after injection with AChR in
Freud's complete adjuvant into the foot pads, the local lymph nodes
were removed. After dissociation, the primed lymphocytes were confronted in vitro with relevant AChR as antigen. In these cultures,
a minor number of lymphocytes transformed to lymphoblasts, which
entered rapid proliferation activity. After a culture period of 3-4
days, the activated lymphoblasts were isolated in discontinuous
Ficoll density gradients, and recultured in the presence of supernatants from Concanavalin A-stimulated mouse spleen cell cultures,
an optimal source of T cell growth factors. These early selected,
"secondary" (2^O), T cell populations were analysed for their functional and phenotypic properties.

    By several criteria, the 2^O anti-AChR lymphocyte populations
were highly enriched antigen specific T cell populations. They
could be reactivated in vitro only in the presence of AChR, and this
antigen had to be presented by syngeneic, MHC-compatible 2^O lymphoid

cells. They had lost the capacity to respond to allogeneic leukocytes in a Mixed Leukocyte Culture. When tested for their proliferative capacity in dilution assays using graded numbers of responder cells in excess of presenter cells and antigen, 2^O anti-AChR populations were shown to be enriched by 100-fold as compared to non-selected, in vivo primed anti-AChR immune lymphoid cells (14). The T cell nature of these cells was established by cytofluorometric analyses using monoclonal antibodies detecting various rat lymphocyte differentiation markers. The 2^O anti-AChR populations expressed markers common to all T cell sublines: they lacked, however, surface immunoglobulins. Ia antigens were not demonstrable in these populations. Among two T cell subline markers, only a T helper cell-specific determinant was detected (15). The T helper nature of 2^O AChR populations was further corroborated by functional studies. Negative evidence was derived from cytotoxicity assays, where 2^O AChR populations were confronted with syngeneic myogenic cells which are known to express abundant doses of AChR. When transferred alone into naive recipient rats, these 2^O AChR cells were in no case able to confer EAMG. In contrast, when transferred along with in vivo primed purified B cells plus AChR/FCA, they facilitated the production of sizeable anti-AChR antibody titers. Recipients treated that way, developed acute EAMG, which correlated with marked subsynaptic mononuclear cell infiltrates (15).

Unexpected results were obtained in analyses of the fine specifity of AChR-specific cells. Both unselected primed as well as 2^O T lymphocytes showed an asymmetric cross-reactivity pattern against AChR derived from Electrophorus, Torpedo and denervated rat muscle. There was no demonstrable crossreactivity between AChR from Torpedo on one side, and Electrophorus or rat on the other. In contrast, AChR-E primed T cells reacted extensively with AChR-R, and vice versa. The crossreactivity between rat and Electrophorus receptors was subsequently used to isolate T populations recognizing Electrophorus plus rat AChR, i.e. autoreactive anti-AChR T cells sensu strictu (14).

Permanent, clonable anti-AChR T cell lines

The previous section dealt with pluriclonal, AChR specific T cell populations. They presumably represent the best cell populations acting in vivo. These populations may be expected to still contain a well balanced repertoire of different AChR-reactive T cell clones with distinct individual antigen receptor properties, as provided by the individual's immune repertoire. Such populations seem to be especially useful for studies of genetic control of immune response repertoires in the pathogenesis.

Other studies will, however, require the establishment of permanent, and possible cloned T cell populations. This is especially

true, when very large numbers of lymphocytos are required, and when
absolute homogeneity of the cell populations is desirable, as in the
case of investigations of idiotypic interactions and molecular studies of antigen receptor interactions. To establish permanent AChR-
specific T cell lines, we used a technique developed by Ben-Nun for
T cell populations recognizing myelin basic protein in Experimental
Autoimmune Encephalomyelitis (16). Two features of this regimen
proved to be vital for the success of line generation. First, the
T line cells had to go through alternating phases of growth promo-
tion. One phase, antigen restimulation, involved antigen presentation by MHC compatible antigen presenter cells (irradiated lymph
node or thymus populations were optimal). Each of these phases had
to be followed by phases of antigen-free propagation cycles, with
the line cells being cultured without any other cellular additives,
but with T cell growth factors instead. It is important to note that
both types of cycles lead to distinct types of cellular activation.
Antigen presentation results in the appearence of large lymphoblasts
which rapidly proliferate (doublication time less than 20 hrs.).
Antigen activated blasts express Ia antigens on their surface. In
contrast, during TCGF propagation, the T cells are gradually reduced
to medium size, they lose their surface Ia, and they proliferate at
rates lower than 1 division per 48 hours.

During the establishment of our permanent AChR-specific T lines,
in most cases we introduced a terminal cell dilution step in early
stages of the line generation. Purified TCGF propagated T line cells
were terminally diluted in the presence of excess antigen and presenter cells. Colonies that grew at clonal cell densities were expanded.

True clonality, i.e. derivation at the expanding inocula from
single cell progenitors, was suggested, though not formally proven
in lines derived from Fl hybrids of Lewis and BN rat strains (Lewis
X BN) Fl. All clonal lines were found to be restricted to antigen
presenter cells of only one parental genotype. So far we did not
detect clones with Fl-specific restriction patterns.

The total of our AChR-specific T cell lines showed fine specificity patterns agreeing with our finding on pluriclonal 2^0 T populations. They were monospecific for the receptor species used for in
vivo priming and in vitro selection. We derived, however, in addition a Fl line which showed a rare cross-reactivity between AChR
from Electrophorus and from Torpedo. Moreover, this cross-reactivity
was only marked when the receptors were presented by Fl presenter
cells.

Obviously, fine specificity patterns of different T clones have
to be analysed in more depth, using defined portions of the AChR
complex. It is expected that such studies will yield information
about structural requirements for the formation of anti-AChR auto-

antibodies, and among them, about the requirement leading to actual disease.

ACKNOWLEDGMENT

This work was supported by grants of Stiftung Volkswagenwerk (to H.W. and I.R.C.) and Deutsche Forschungsgemeinschaft (to H.W.).

REFERENCES

1. Engel, A.G., Lambert, E.H. and Howard F.H., Mayo Clin. Proc. 52:267-280 (1977).
2. Toyka, K.V., Drachman, D.B., Pestronk, A. and Kao, I., Science 190:397-399 (1975).
3. Appel, S.H., Anwyl, R., Mc Adams, M.W. and Elias, S., Proc. Nat. Sci. 74:2130-2134 (1977).
4. Feltkamp, T.E.W., Van Den Berg-Loonen, P.M., Nijenhuis, L.E., Engelfriet, C.P., Van Rossum, A.L., Van Loghem, J.J. and Osterhuis, H.J.G.H., Br. Med. J. i:131-133 (1974).
5. McDevitt, H.O., N. Eng. J. Med. 303:1514-1517 (1980).
6. Conti-Tronconi, B.M., Morgutti, B.M., Sgirlanzoni, A. and Clementi, F., Neurol. 29:496-501 (1979).
7. Abramsky, O., Aharonov, A., Webb, C. and Fuchs, S., Clin. Exp. Immunol. 19:11-16 (1975).
8. Lefvert, A.K., Bergström, K., Scand. J. Immunol. 813:115-119 (1978).
9. Cantor, H., Boyse, E.A., Cold Spring Harbor Symp. Quant Biol. 41:23-32 (1977).
10. Wekerle, H.R., Hohlfeld, U.P., Ketelson, J.R., Ketelson, J.R., Kalies, I., Ann. N. Y. Acad. Sci. 377:455-476 (1981).
11. Wekerle, H., J. Exp. Med. 147:233-250 (1978).
12. Wekerle, H. and Begemann, M., J. Immunol. 116:159-164 (1976).
13. Wekerle, H., Ben-Nun, A., Hurtenbach, U. and Prester, M., in: "Genetic Control of Autoimmunity", Rose, N.R., Warner, N.L. and Bigazzi, P. (Eds.), Academic Press, New York, pp. 413-432 (1978).
14. Hohlfeld, R., Kalies, I., Heinz, F., Kalden, J.R. and Wekerle, H, J. Immunol. 126:1355-1359 (1981).
15. Hohlfeld, R., Kalies, I., Ernst, M., Ketelson, U.P. and Wekerle, H., J. Neurol. Sci. (in press).
16. Ben-Nun, A., Wekerle, H. and Cohen, I.R., Eur. J. Immunol. 11:195-199 (1981).

HUMAN IgG SHORT-TERM SENSITIZING ANAPHYLACTIC ANTIBODY:

DIFFERENCES IN PROPERTIES FROM THOSE OF IgG$_4$

W.E. Parish

Environmental Safety Laboratory
Unilever Research, Colworth House
Sharnbrook, Bedford, MK44 1LQ, United Kingdom

Two anaphylactic antibodies are found in human sera. IgE, the classical reaginic antibody which occurs in very small amounts, which passively sensitizes human skin in vivo for four weeks or longer, and the passive sensitizing property is susceptible to heating at 56°C or treatment with reducing chemicals. The other antibody with anaphylactic or very similar properties is part of the total IgG, and at present is known as IgG S-TS, or short-term sensitizing, because it sensitizes human or monkey skin for 2 to 4 hours only. The passive sensitizing property of IgG S-TS resists heating at 56°C and resists treatment with reducing chemicals.

Properties of IgG S-TS

The properties of IgG S-TS (1-4) are:

1. The antibody is present in pure fractions of IgG, uncontaminated by IgE.
2. On injection into the skin of man or monkey, the IgG antibody sensitizes the site for 2 to 4 hours only. The titre in passive cutaneous anaphylaxis tests is low, not greater than a 1/16 dilution.
3. IgG fractions containing S-TS activity will partially block sensitization by IgE for about 4 hours, but as pure preparations of IgG S-TS are not available the impeding or blocking activity cannot be attributed to IgG S-TS.
4. IgG S-TS binds weakly to tissues and is easily eluted from preparations of lung and skin in vitro by washing.
5. IgG in fractions containing S-TS activity binds to purified preparations of human basophils in vitro. Treatment of the baso-

211

phils with monospecific anti-IgG (γ) releases significant amounts
of histamine. Treatment with the specific antigen does not.

6. The ability to sensitize tissue is unaffected by heating the
    serum at 56°C or 60°C for up to 4 hours.

7. Sensitizing ability also resists chemical reduction with 0.1M
    2-mercapto-ethanol which inactivates IgE.

8. The skin responses in vivo in monkeys can be differentiated from
    immune complex-mediated (Arthus) reactions because depletion of
    complement and of neutrophils, both essential for Arthus reac-
    tions, do not diminsh IgG S-TS responses. Some variations in
    results of the complement-depletion tests are attributed to
    technique and sources of reagents.

9. Though IgG S-TS tends to occur in sera containing IgG precipi-
    tins, many (over 300) sera containing IgG complement-activating
    antibodies to milk, egg, horse serum, streptococcal exotoxins,
    Aspergillus or Micropolyspore faeni (farmers lung) have no S-TS
    activity. The sensitizing activity is therefore not a property
    of complement-activating precipitins.

Detection

The only means of detection, at present, is by passive transfer
of serum to man in Prausnitz-Kustner-type tests, or to monkeys in
passive cutaneous anaphylaxis procedures. This is likely to continue
until the particular immunoglobulin subclass is defined, related to
its biological activity. It would appear that not all the molecules
of one immunoglobulin subclass have identical biological activity.

Passive transfer tests in man have a serious disadvantage in the
potential hazard of transferring viral infection, particularly hepatitis virus, for which the donor sera should be examined before the
test. Sera need to be heated at 56°C for one or two hours, or passed
down an anti-IgE insoluble immuno-adsorbent column to remove any IgE
antibody sensitization, and subsequently sterilised by a small
volume Millipore filter attached to a syringe to remove any bacteria. Challenge of the sites treated with the test serum, may be by
prick test, or intracutaneous injection of 0.05 ml of a nonirritant,
nonhistamine-releasing concentration of the antigen.

The response in human skin sensitized by IgG S-TS is slightly
slower to appear than that in sites sensitized by IgE, and usually
much weaker. There is a discrete weal without pseudopodia, and an
irregular surrounding flare. It also itches less than that of IgE
responses to the same antigen tested at the same time, but after
24 hours sensitization instead of the 2 or 4 hours of IgG S-TS.

The method usually used to detect IgG S-TS is passive cutaneous
anaphylaxis in monkeys. This avoids the potential hazard of transfer
of infection to man. The procedure is a little less sensitive than

the test on man, but not as much as the tenfold difference sometimes observed between man and monkey in tests for IgE sensitization. Sera are injected into the skin of monkeys in 0.1 ml volume, and challenge is made at about two or four hours later. The blue indicator dye is injected ten minutes before challenge, to identify any sera which may have induced histamine release or increased vascular permeability, and these are excluded from the results of the subsequent treatment with antigen. Antigen may be administered by intravenous injection, with a further small amount of dye if necessary, or in an appropriate concentration by intracutaneous injection of 0.05 ml over each test site with relevant controls. Intracutaneous injection results in stronger reactions than seen following intravenous challenge.

The site of a positive response may appear as a circumscribed dense blue area, about 10 mm diameter, or more frequently as a blue ring about 15 mm diameter with a pale centre. The pale centre is believed to result from the blocking activity of IgG not specific for the antigen, because mixtures of IgG S-TS with other IgG increase the size of the pale centre, and conversely, dilution of the IgG S-TS containing serum or fraction resulted in the homogeneous dense blue responses. The titre of positive sera was invariably weak, seldom above 1/16.

At present the human PK or monkey PCA tests remain more reliable than in vitro tests of passive sensitization of human or monkey lung or skin. Not all samples of lung can be sensitized by IgG S-TS in vitro, and though skin may be more readily sensitized, the response on antigenic challenge, histamine and eosinophil chemotactic factor release is much less than that released by IgE mediated reactions.

Inhibition of IgE-mediated PCA by IgG preparations containing IgG S-TS

IgE non-specific for a test antigen, in sufficient amount blocks sensitization of skin by IgE antigen-specific antibody. IgG fractions containing IgG S-TS were therefore examined for their potential to block sensitization by IgE as has been described for myeloma IgG$_4$ (5,6), and to block sensitization by IgG S-TS of another antigen specificity.

Preparations of IgG, or of IgG containing S-TS activity, (both adsorbed to remove all IgE) were examined for their ability to impede or block sensitization by IgE antibody. The test IgE antibody preparation was adsorbed to remove nearly all the IgG, and it has a monkey PCA titre of 256 on challenge 24 hours after sensitization. The normal IgG or IgG S-TS preparations were injected into the monkey skin followed at intervals by injection of the IgE antibody into the same sites and subsequently challenged with antigen at 2 hours, or 4 hours, or 24 hours.

IgG from a normal person, at 50µg concentration reduced the IgE
PCA titre from 256 to 64 at 2 and 4 hours, and at 100µg to a titre
of 32 at 2 hours challenge. This showed that normal IgG, in excess
or unphysiological amount, could for a short time reduce the sensitizing potential of IgE antibody.

In contrast a preparation of IgG anti-tetanus, containing S-TS
activity, at only 10µg concentration reduced IgE PCA titre to 64
at 2 and 4 hours, and at 50µg concentration reduced the IgE PCA titre
to 16 at 2 hours, and to 32 at 4 hours after sensitization by IgE.
None of the IgG preparations impeded IgE sensitization at the 24
hour time of antigenic challenge. Therefore IgG S-TS, or another
component in the preparation (which contained some IgG_4) had greater
short-term impeding properties for IgE sensitization than did normal
(non allergenic) IgG.

Incidence of IgG S-TS activity

The overall incidence of detection of IgG S-TS antibodies, or
heat-stable short-term sensitizing antibodies presumably IgG S-TS
is 6 to 7% of the sera examined, most of which are from allergic
persons. In some groups of patients the incidence of detection of
heat-stable antibody is as high as 30% to 50% (7) but this results
from a combination of the selection procedure, and possibly the
nature of the antigen, e.g. aspergillus and budgerigar which appear
to induce both anaphylactic sensitivity and formation of IgG preci-
pitins.

The anaphylactic IgG antibody has been detected in the sera of
normal i.e. clinically non-allergic persons, but who react to antigen by prick test or by intracutaneous injection. These persons
usually have appreciable amounts of IgG antibody to the antigen,
but may have very little IgE antibody, below the amount considered
significant to the same antigen, and below the amount able to confer
anaphylactic sensitivity on monkey or human skin.

IgG S-TS in clinical disorders

IgG S-TS, or heat-stable short-term sensitizing antibodies presumably IgG S-TS, have been reported in a wide range of clinical
disorders which are manifestations of anaphylactic sensitivity. The
clinical examples of IgG S-TS association may be considered in three
main groups, a result of injected antigens, gastro-intestinal food
allergy and in asthma. Examples of each are cited here, but a more
complete review is available (4).

Injected substances. As IgG S-TS forms part of the total IgG, it is not surprising that the stimulation of much IgG by some substances should not also include some IgG S-TS. Tetanus toxoid and therapeutic horse gamma globulin stimulate formation of IgG S-TS (2). Protamine sulphate was found to induce formation of an IgG antibody with apparent anaphylactic properties, though this appeared to be complement dependent (8). Another drug found to induce formation of IgG anaphylactic antibody is Succinylcholine. In examination of five cases of anaphylactic sensitivity to this drug by PK passive transfer, the sera of three had IgE antibody, and in one of them there was also a heat-stable IgG anaphylactic antibody (9).

Gastro-intestinal food allergy. IgG S-TS is found in patients with food allergy manifested as gastro-intestinal changes or asthma. The IgG antibody is found more frequently than IgE in patients whose intestinal signs are delayed several hours after exposure to the food antigen. Milk, especially β-lactoglobulin is the most frequently detected antigen (1,2,10). Other food antigens are egg and wheat.

Asthma. A great diversity of antigens have been found to induce asthma associated with IgG S-TS antibody, some cases of which have been confirmed by inhalation provocation tests. The antigens include house dust mite (11,12), house dust (13), grass pollen, milk, egg and budgerigar (7), and platinum (14).

In some patients no clinical difference was observed in patients whose asthma was assocated with IgE or IgG S-TS, but in one study nine patients with cryptogenic (intrinsic) asthma characerised by "late age of onset" and negative prick tests to twenty two routine common allergens, four had heat-stable short-term sensitizing antibodies and no IgE (7). This is not certain evidence that IgG S-TS is a major mediator of cryptogenic asthma, but the findings indicate that this antibody may be a significant mediator of asthma in non atopic persons.

IgG S-TS is not a property of IgG4. The IgG subclass or subclasses of IgG S-TS have not been identified. There is strong evidence that it is not IgG_1, and as this is a subclass activating complement, it affords further support that IgG S-TS is independent of the direct action of complement. Moreover, there is no evidence that IgG S-TS activity is mediated by IgG_4, and no definite support for some assertions that IgG_4 is an anaphylactic antibody.

There are some associations between IgG S-TS and IgG_4. IgG S-TS and increased amounts of IgG_4 tend to occur together in sera of allergic persons. IgG fractions containing IgG S-TS and myeloma IgG_4 reduce monkey PCA by IgE for about 4 hours. Furthermore, IgG containing S-TS and IgG_4 bind to human basophils, but do not sensitize them anaphylactically to antigen.

Our evidence that IgG$_4$ is not an anaphylactic antibody is as follows:

1. There is no consistent relation between the amount of total and allergen-specific IgG$_4$ and IgG S-TS activity. Though increased amounts of IgG$_4$ and IgG S-TS tend to occur together, frequently with increased amounts of IgE antibody, in the sera of allergic persons, there are several instances in which there is almost no IgG$_4$ antibody to the antigen in sera containing IgG S-TS activity.

    Many sera with normal or increased amounts of total IgG$_4$, and with significant amounts of IgG$_4$ to a particular antigen do not confer PCA sensitivity in monkeys for two or four hours.

    Purified preparations of IgG$_4$ did not confer PCA sensitivity in monkeys. Complexes of IgG$_4$ and specific antigen, and heat-aggregated IgG$_4$ did not induce significant increased vascular permeability in monkeys.

2. Treatment of human lung preparations, shown to be susceptible to sensitization in vitro by S-TS and by IgE were not sensitized by sera containing IgG$_4$ to release histamine on exposure to the relevant antigen.

3. Leucocyte suspensions, containing basophils, prepared from eight persons with total amounts of IgG$_4$ of 0.45, 0.55, 0.6, 0.7, 0.8, 1.1 and 1.35 mg/ml did not release significant amounts of histamine when treated with anti-IgG$_4$. Results of challenge with relevant antigens were not attributable to IgG$_4$ because most of the persons also had IgE antibody.

4. Whole (intact) serum containing 0.8 mg/ml IgG$_4$ did not sensitize human basophils to release histamine on subsequent treatment with anti-IgG$_4$ or with the relevant antigen. Separation of total IgG$_4$ (5.6 mg/ml) and of antigen (egg) specific IgG$_4$ (2.4 mg/ml) by immuno-adsorption techniques, provided samples for treatment of human basophils. These sensitized the cells to release histamine when tested with anti-IgG$_4$ but not on testing with the specific antigen. These purified preparations contained more IgG$_4$ than those to which cells would be exposed in vivo, and did not contain any of the other plasma proteins that may compete with IgG$_4$ in vivo.

    Features of the test detecting IgG$_4$ -Anti-IgG$_4$ histamine release were

    a. Histamine release was observed most readily in cells which released significant amounts of histamine on treatment with IgE followed by anti-IgE. (Samples that released significant amounts of histamine spontaneously were discarded).

b. No significant net amount of histamine was released in the cells treated with IgG_1 and anti-IgG_1

    with IgG_1 and anti-IgG_4

    with IgG_4 and diluted normal rabbit IgG

    with IgG_4 and anti-IgG_1

Attempts to remove the anti-IgG_4 antibody by immuno-adsorption with IgG_4 resulted in a product that caused spontaneous release of histamine, but this was not evidence, per se, of stimulation of the cells by immune complexes.

c. The histamine release from cells treated with IgG_4 followed by anti-IgG_4 occurred with dilute solutions of anti-IgG_4 and not by stronger concentrations. Histamine release could also be induced by anti IgG_4 $F(ab)_2$.

The binding of IgG_4 to the leucocytes was stable for the duration of the test.

5. IgG_4 at 2.5 mg/ml impeded sensitization of human basophils by IgE. This was observed particularly in tests with small amounts of IgE antibody. There was less or no blocking if stronger preparations of IgE antibody were used. The impeding effect was reduced after 15 minutes. The effect was dose-time related and was considered to be weak. There was no evidence that IgG_4 and IgE competed for the same receptors; the effect appeared to be due to stereohindrance by the IgG_4 blocking the reactions of the antigen with IgE. IgE was taken up by the cells during the period of exposure; in previous tests there was no evidence that any bound IgG_4 was eluted.

Conclusions

It is concluded from the above data that IgG S-TS activity is not a property of IgG_4 in the sera examined. There is no evidence in any test that monkey skin in vivo or tissues in vitro treated with IgG_4 show anaphylactic change on subsequent challenge with antigen. However, IgG_4 has some tissue-binding properties similar to those of anaphylactic antibodies. Myeloma IgG_4 has been reported to impede sensitization of monkey skin by IgE for a few hours, as do preparations containing IgG S-TS. Furthermore, IgG_4 separated from serum will bind to basophils, making them susceptible to histamine release on challenge with anti-IgG_4, and will weakly impede sensitization by IgE. However, IgG_4 in intact serum does not have this property, so the significance of the basophil binding in vivo is doubtful.

REFERENCES

1. Parish, W.E., Lancet ii:591 (1970).
2. Parish, W.E., in: "Asthma, Physiology, Immunopharmacology and Treatment" (Eds. K.F. Austen and L.M. Lichtenstein), p. 71, Academic Press, New York (1973).
3. Parish, W.E., in: "Immediate Hypersensitivity; modern concepts and developments" (Ed. by M.K. Bach), p. 277, Marcel Dekker, New York (1978).
4. Parish, W.E., Brit. J. Dermatol. 105:223 (1981).
5. Stanworth, D.R. and Smith, A.K., Clin. Allergy 3:37 (1973).
6. Vijay, H.M. and Perelmutter, L., Internat. Arch. Allergy Appl. Immunol. 53:78 (1977).
7. Pepys, J., Parish, W.E., Stenius-Aarniala, B. and Wide, L., Clin. Allergy 9:645 (1979).
8. Lakin, J.D., Blocker, T.J., Strong, M. and Yocum, W., Allergy Clin. Immunol. 61:102 (1978).
9. Moneret-Vautrin, D.A., Laxenaire, M.C. and Moeller, R., Clin. Allergy 11:175 (1981).
10. Brighton, W.D., Clin. Allergy 10:97 (1980).
11. Bryant, D.H., Burns, M.W. and Lazarus, L., Brit. Med. J. iv:589 (1973).
12. Bryant, D.H., Burns, M.W. and Lazarus, L., Allergy and Clin. Immunol. 56:417 (1975).
13. Berry, J.B. and Brighton, W.D., Clin. Allergy 7:401 (1977).
14. Pepys, J., Parish, W.E., Cromwell, O. and Hughes, E.G., Clin. Allergy 9:99 (1979).

LEUKOTRIENES AND LIPID FACTORS: MEDIATORS AND

MODULATORS OF THE INFLAMMATORY REACTIONS

W. König,[1] K.D. Bremm,[1] K. Theobald,[1] Ph. Pfeiffer,[1]
B. Szperalski,[1] A. Bohn,[1] P. Borgeat,[2] B. Spur,[3]
A.E.G. Crea,[3] and G. Falsone[3]

Lehrstuhl Med. Mikrobiologie und Immunologie
Ruhr-Universität Bochum, FRG[1]; Département
d'Endocrinologie Moléculaire, Le Centre de L-Université
Laval, SteFoye, Québec Canada[2]; Institut für organische
Chemie, Universität Düsseldorf, FRG[3]

In the past years the immunological and chemical analysis of
mediators involved in inflammation has led to a remarkable change
in the understanding of allergic and inflammatory reactions. The
discovery of the IgE-immunoglobulin as the antibody molecule inducing
immediate type hypersensitivity reactions as well as the molecular
analysis of the anaphylatoxins (C3a, C5a) emphasized the major role
of the mast cells in allergic and inflammatory disease processes.
Mast cell activation by immunological and non immunological mechanisms led to the release of preformed and newly generated mediators (1). Among those were products previously called "slow reacting
substance" (SRS), lipid chemotactic factor (ECF) and platelet activating factor (PAF=AGEPC). Only recently the chemical structures of
these molecules have been established (2-5). Evidence was also presented in the seventies that in addition to mast cells secondary
cells of inflammation such as neutrophils, mononuclear cells and
macrophages released mediators which previously had been solely
attributed to the mast cell alone (6,7). Thus, the concept of the
interdependency of various cells in inflammatory reactions initiated
by low molecular weight mediators was established.

Polyunsaturated fatty acids play a role as precursors of biologically active compounds that can act as mediators or modulators
of various cell functions. Three main groups of derivaties -the
prostaglandins, the thromboxanes and the recently discovered
leukotrienes- are formed by oxygenation and further transformation

219

of various polyunsaturated fatty acids of which arachidonic acid
plays the most significant role (8). Among the lipoxygenase transformation products are factors with pronounced effect on leukocyte
migration and vascular permeability; the biological activity referred for forty years as slow reacting substance of anaphylaxis is
comprised of three related metabolites of arachidonic acid LTC_4, D_4
and E_4. The recent synthesis of these compounds has permitted an
insight into the biological and stereospecific requirements for
their cellular interactions.

INDUCTION, BIOLOGICAL AND CHEMICAL CHARACTERIZATION OF
LIPOXYGENASE TRANSFORMATION PRODUCTS

As early as 1975 we presented evidence that a non preformed
mediator assayed by the Boyden chamber technique with guinea pig and
human eosinophils was generated on stimulation of human PMN, eosinophils, mononuclear cells, basophils as well as rat mast cells. This
factor was named ECF since unlike guinea pig neutrophils obtained
by casein injection it demonstrated a pronounced chemotactic activity for the guinea pig eosinophil (6,7). The observation that preformed eosinophil chemotactic activity (termed tetrapeptide ECF-A)
was minimal compared to the chemotactic activity obtained after
stimulation of cells led us to further analyze the ECF activity.
When human PMNs were incubated with the calcium-ionophore A 23 187
and the supernatants were assayed for chemotactic activity it was
demonstrated that chemotactic activity appeared and decreased at
later times of secretion. The chemotactic activity preceded the
secretion of granular and microsomal enzymes (9). Similar findings
were obtained when the cells were stimulated with opsonized zymosan
or antigen-antibody complexes. By subcellular fractionation studies
it became apparent that the chemotactic factor activity was derived
from the plasma membrane (10). These results were confirmed when we
described the chemotactic factor formation on incubation of the
cells such as human PMNs, mononuclear cells, rat basophilic leu-
kaemia cells with arachidonic acid (11). With the observation that
arachidonic acid was able to generate lipid chemotactic factor
activity the question arose for the common cell-biological link in
the course of cell activation leading to ECF-production.

Both stimuli -the calcium ionophore and opsonized zymosan- as
well as melittin lead to cell triggering resulting in the activation
of phospholipase A_2 with the subsequent formation of arachidonic acid
from the various phospholipids. We suggested that the generation of
lipid chemotactic factor activity proceeds via the conversion of
arachidonic acid by a lipoxygenase like enzyme within the cytosol
which, assayed with guinea pig eosinophils, attracted these
cells (12). The chemical identification of the lipoxygenase transformation products has provided a more precise understanding of the
results obtained from the various biological models. All classes of

leukocytes possess both 5-lipoxgenase and 15-lipoxygenase activities
that transform arachidonic acid to mono- and di-HETEs and the more
complex products such as the peptide lipid conjugates LTC$_4$ and LTD$_4$.
LTB$_4$ (5 (S), 12 (R) dihydroxy-6, 14 cis-8, 10 transeicosatetraenoic
acid) is formed following an initial lipoxygenase attack at position
C5 on the arachidonic acid molecule (Fig.1). Molecular oxygen is
inserted to produce the unstable intermediate 5-hydroxy-peroxy-
eicosatetraenoic acid (5-HPETE). This compound may be converted
either to the corresponding monohydroxy fatty acid via the glu-
tathionine peroxidase system or to another unstable intermediate
leukotriene A4. The term leukotrienes was proposed by Samuelsson for
these compounds to indicate that they were derived from leukocytes
and that they possessed a conjugated triene structure (8). Hydroly-
sis of LTA$_4$ leads to the formation of 5, 12 dihydroxy fatty acid and
isomers. The structure for LTB$_4$ was identified by Borgeat and
Samuelsson (2). In cooperation with Borgeat we analyzed the ECF
containing supernatants obtained after ionophore and melittin stimulation. When ^{14}C labelled PMN were stimulated and the chemotactic
factor activity containing supernatant was subjected to thin layer
chromatography and autoradiography multiple spots were identified.
Among them were spots with an Rf value identical to LTB$_4$ and additional mono-HETE. Also the incubation of 5-HETE with ^{14}C labelled
platelets induced the generation of 12-HETE suggesting that mono-
HETEs may interact interdependently with the various cell sources.
These data were confirmed by reversed phase HPLC. The analysis of
mono- and di-HETEs with regard to their eosinophil chemotactic properties revealed that LTB$_4$ exerted the most pronounced effects
towards eosinophils (13). As to the activity of LTB$_4$ and its isomers
towards human PMNs the data of Ford-Hutchinson and Goetzl et. al.
are confirmed (14, 15). Among the di-HETEs, LTB$_4$ is the most active
factor at a range of 10^{-7} -10^{-9}M, while the 5 (S), 12 (S) di-HETE
is less active by 10-100 fold. Injection of the various HETEs into
the peritoneal cavity of rats led to a substantial change in the
distribution of the cells. The peritoneal cells of control animals
are comprised of 5-10% mast cells, 4-8% eosinophils, 0-2% PMN and
75-80% peritoneal cells. A significant influx of eosinophils and
neutrophils is observed with LTB$_4$. There is no evidence that there
is a selective activity of the mono- or di- HETE for the neutrophil
or eosinophil alone. LTB$_4$ was also injected into the guinea pig
skin and the influx of cells was examined during various times. Ten
min. after injection a marked increase of granulocytes (eosinophils,
neutrophils) is observed; after 30 min. these cells were distributed
in the adjacent tissue. Two hrs. after injection the cells slowly
disappeared. Indeed, as has been recently described, eosinophils
by themselves produce mono- and di-HETEs on stimulation with the
calcium ionophore (16). These results confirm our published data
that eosinophils on incubation with the ionophore generate lipid
chemotactic factor activity for eosinophils (ECF) (6).

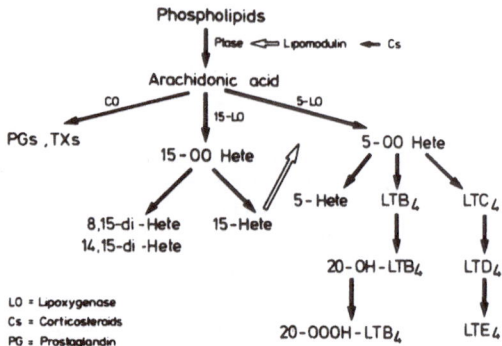

Fig. 1.   Generation and transformation of arachidonic acid by the
          5-lipoxygenase and cyclooxygenase enzyme.

        Conjugation of LTA_4 by a glutathionine-S-transferase enzyme
leads to the production of LTC_4. On exposure to γ-glutamyltranspep-
tidase LTD_4 is generated which after removal of the glycine residue
is converted to LTE_4. The unique capacity of this mediator class to
preferentially impair pulmonary compliance compared to conductance
was confirmed by administration of LTC_4 and LTD_4 in guinea pigs and
humans. Leukotrienes as well as PAF in contrast to the synthetic
leukotriene methylesters also change the vascular permeability.

MODULATION OF INFLAMMATORY REACTIONS BY LIPID FACTORS

        Endogenous HETEs are not only mediators of inflammation. They
also modulate the responsiveness of granulocytes in the presence of
C5a. Eosinophils in the presence or absence of the various mono-
and di-HETEs were stimulated with C5a at a sub-optimal concentration. Our data indicate that addition of endogeneous HETEs to the
cells induce a pronounced chemokinetic activation of the cells. The
fact that an intermediate response is observed with LTB_4, the all
trans isomers of LTB_4, 12-HETE and 5-HETE when present in the upper
and lower compartment of the Boyden chamber can be attributed to
the fact that these compounds deactivate the cells for a further
response towards C5a. It also emphasizes that the mono- and di-HETEs
exert profound chemokinetic properties and thus modulate the responsiveness of the cells towards other chemoattractants.

        The biological role of the platelet activating factor (PAF=
AGEPC) as a newly generated mediator of inflammation has been ap-
preciated in the past and facilitated quite recently by the chemical
analysis and synthesis of this molecule (3, 5). AGEPC and related
phospholipids are released by many types of leukocytes. The relative
quantities of PAF produced and the preferential stimuli may vary for
the different types of leukocytes. Basophils, monocytes and macro-

phages appear to generate greater amounts of PAF than neutrophils, eosinophils or mast cells. We studied the effect of the C5a induced eosinophil and neutrophil chemotaxis in the absence or presence of synthetic PAF or structural analogues. PAF was either present in the upper compartment with the cells or in the lower compartment with C5a. Incubation of cells in the presence of PAF or analogues and subsequent stimulation with C5a leads to a more pronounced modulation of the chemotactic responsiveness as compared to experiments in which C5a and PAF or structural analogues are present in the lower compartment of the chamber. These results again stress that lipid mediators may modulate the responsiveness of the cells towards peptide chemoattractants. In the C5a induced contraction of the guinea pig ileum PAF leads to an enhanced contractile response while structural analogues often inhibited the response.

We also studied the anti-IgE and allergen induced histamine release from human basophils and demonstrated a donor dependent enhancement with mono-HETEs (5 HPETE, 5-HETE, 12-HETE) as well as with LTC_4, D_4 and E_4 while the leukotriene methylesters were ineffective. These results combined suggest that lipoxygenase factors generated by various stimulation of the cells modulate the responsiveness of these cells. The data also emphasize that lipid factors serve as obligatory components in transducing membrane signals via receptor ligand interactions. To probe this assumption a membrane biochemical model of cell activation was suggested. On addition of polienoic and polynoic acids the anti-IgE or ionophore induced histamine release was studied. It was observed that the addition of polienoic and poliynoic acids markedly inhibited the histamine release. The 4,7,10,13 poliynoic acid proved to be the most potent inhibitor. We also studied the generation of lipid chemotactic factor activity (ECF) in the presence of the arachidonic acid analogues on stimulation of the cells with the ionophore or melittin. Again, it is demonstrated that 4,7,10,13 poliynoic acid was the most potent inhibitor (1). These data were also confirmed when subcellular fractions containing 5, 15 lipoxygenase activity were studied as has been described. A further model in which the phospholipase-arachidonic acid sequence as a common link for cell membrane activation was studied, referred to the C5a induced contraction of smooth muscle as well as histamine release from mast cells. With arachidonic acid analogues a potent inhibition was obtained.

CONCLUSION

The biological potency of the lipoxygenase mediators has been by now clearly established. Our experimental studies over the past seven years cover the generation of a lipid chemotactic factor which, assayed primarily with guinea pig eosinophils, proved to be chemotactic and was termed ECF. A further analysis of the various stimuli inducing lipid chemotactic factor activity led us to suggest the phospholipase-arachidonic acid sequence as a common link of cell membrane activation. These data were confirmed with endogeneous and synthetic mono- and di-HETEs as well as by immunopharmacological studies using arachidonic acid analogues. It became also apparent that these factors modulate the responsiveness of the cells towards other stimuli and are obligatory components in transducing membrane signals transformed by various immunological stimuli. These data clearly indicate that structural analogues as well as the interference with the lipoxygenase and/or cyclooxygenase pathway will serve as a potential immunopharmacological tool to counteract inflammatory disease processes.

REFERENCES

1. König, W., Pfeiffer, P., Szperalski, B. and Bohn, A., in "Behring Institute Mitteilungen", 68:30-50 (1981).
2. Borgeat, P. and Samuelsson, B., J. Biol. Chem. 254:7865-7869 (1979).
3. Benveniste, J., Camussi, J. and Polonsky, J., Allergy 12:138-142 (1977).
4. Corey, E.J., Clark, D.A., Goto, G., Marfat, A., Mioskowski, C., Samuelsson, B. and Hammarström, S., J. Am. Chem. Soc. 102:1436-1439 (1980).
5. Demopoulos, C.A., Pinckard, R.N. and Hanahan, D.J., J. Biol. Chem. 254:9355-9358 (1979).
6. Czarnetzki, B.M., König, W. and Lichtenstein, L.M., J. Immunol. 117:229-234 (1976).
7. König, W., Czarnetzki, B.M. and Lichtenstein, L.M., J. Immunol. 117:235-246 (1976).
8. Samuelsson, B., "Trends in Pharmacological Sciences", pp. 227-230 (1980).
9. König, W., Frickhofen, N. and Tesch, H., Immunology 36:733-742 (1979).
10. Frickhofen, N. and König, W., Immunology 37:111-122 (1979).
11. König, W., Tesch, H. and Frickhofen, N., Eur. J. Immunol. 8:434-437 (1978).
12. Tesch, H. and König, W., Scand. J. Immunol. 11:409-418 (1980).
13. König, W., Kunau, H.W. and Borgeat, P., in: "Leukotrienes and other Lipoxygenase Products", Samuelsson, B. and Paoletti, R. (eds), Vol.9, pp. 301-314 Raven Press, New York (1982).
14. Ford-Hutchinson, A.W., J. Royal Soc. Med. 74:831-833 (1981).
15. Goetzl, E.J. and Pickett, W.C., J. Exp. Med., 153:482-487 (1981).
16. Jörg, A., Henderson, W.R., Murphy, R.C. and Klebanoff, J., J. Exp. Med. 155:390-402 (1982).

CALMODULIN AND HUMAN INFLAMMATORY REACTIONS

G. Marone, M. Columbo, S. Poto,
P. Bianco, and M. Condorelli

University of Naples II School of Medicine
Department of Medicine
80131 Naples, Italy

Calmodulin is a low-molecular-weight Ca^{2+}-binding protein, which influences numerous Ca^{2+}-mediated intracellular processes in a variety of tissues and is thus considered to be an important regulator of cellular metabolism (1,2). The presence of calmodulin has been demonstrated in human (3) and animal leukocytes (4,5). This protein controls a variety of enzymes including cyclic AMP phosphodiesterase (6), adenylate cyclase (7) and phospholipase A_2 (8,9). Calmodulin may also be involved in the regulation of microtubular assembly and disassembly (10,11).

Inflammatory reactions in man are characterized by the release of chemical mediators from basophils, polymorphonuclear leukocytes (PMNs), and platelets, following immunological activation (12,13). Therefore, the biochemical and pharmacological control of these release reactions is important in controlling immunological processes. We have shown that histamine secretion from human basophils is modulated by intracellular Ca^{2+} (13) and cylic AMP (14), the state of microtubule assembly, and the activation of phospholipase A_2 (15). More recently, it has been shown that the release of lysosomal enzymes from human PMNs is also controlled by intracellular cyclic AMP (16), the state of microtubule assembly, and probably the activation of phospholipase A_2 (17).

Several calmodulin antagonists which bind to calmodulin and selectively inhibit Ca^{2+}-calmodulin-induced activation of enzymes have been identified. Trifluoperazine dihydrochloride (TFP) and the sulfonamide derivative N-(6-aminohexyl)-5-chloro-1-napthalene sulfonamide (W-7) have been reported to bind selectively to calmodulin (18,19).

We have recently performed a series of experiments to investigate the possible role of calmodulin in inflammation by evaluating the effects of several calmodulin antagonists on histamine release from basophils, enzyme release from PMNs, and on platelet aggregation.

TFP, at low concentration (1-20 uM), binds to calmodulin with high affinity and is a potent and highly specific inhibitor of calmodulin-mediated processes (18,20). TFP inhibits calmodulin stimulation of phosphodiesterase (21) and adenylate cyclase (7) inactivates calmodulin regulation of smooth muscle contraction (22) and phospholipase A_2 activity (8).

We tested the effect of TFP on histamine secretion from human basophils induced by immunological (antigen and anti-IgE) and non-immunological (f-met-peptide and the Ca^{2+} ionophore A23187) stimuli. Figure 1 shows that TFP produces a concentration-dependent inhibition of histamine release by human basophils stimulated by both Group I Rye grass antigen and anti-IgE. Similar results were obtained when the cells were pretreated with TFP and then challenged with non-immunological stimuli such as f-met-peptide or the Ca^{2+} ionophore A23187. In these experiments, the cells were pretreated for 2 minutes with TFP before the addition of the stimuli. Incubation times longer than 3 minutes at $3x10^{-5}M$ TFP or concentrations equal to or larger than $5x10^{-5}M$ were found to cause leakage of the cell's content of lactate dehydrogenase into the extracellular medium.

To test the specificity of this observation, we have shown that TFP sulfoxide, which has very low affinity to calmodulin (18), is practically ineffective to inhibit histamine secretion from human basophils (Figure 1). The minimal effect of TFP sulfoxide on histamine secretion emphasizes both the specificity of the effect and the potential involvement of calmodulin in the release process.

To extend the observation described above, we have examined the effect of another specific calmodulin antagonist, W-7, which has been extensively characterized by Hidaka et al. (19,23). They have shown that W-7 selectively binds to calmodulin and inhibits several calmodulin-dependent enzymes (24) and cellular functions (23,25). We have found that W-7 inhibits, in a dose-dependent manner, the histamine secretion induced by antigen, anti-IgE, f-met-peptide, and the Ca^{2+} ionophore A23187.

The release of lysosomal enzymes from human PMNs is a pivoting event in human inflammatory processes. Recently, we have investigated the possible role of calmodulin on enzyme release from human PMNs by evaluating first the intracellular concentration of this protein and second the effects of two specific inhibitors of calmodulin, such as TFP and W-7. Calmodulin was assayed by a specific radioimmunoassay in highly purified PMNs ($\cong$ 99%). Human PMN was

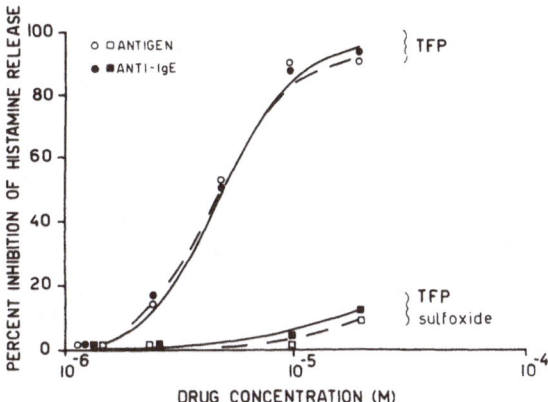

Fig. 1.   Dose response curves of inhibition of antigen and anti-IgE-
induced histamine release from human basophils by trifluoperazine dihydrochloride (TFP) and trifluoperazine
sulfoxide.

found to contain approximately 3×10^6 molecules of calmodulin equal
to approximately 0.03% of the total cellular protein. We have also
confirmed the presence of this protein in human PMNs by indirect immunofluorescent studies using a monospecific sheep anti-calmodulin
antibody. We also found that W-7, a specific calmodulin inhibitor,
blocks lysosomal enzyme release from PMNs. The β-glucuronidase and
lysozyme release from human PMNs induced by several immunological
(C_{5a}, serum-treated Zymosan, Concanavalin A, etc.) and non-immunological stimuli, was inhibited by W-7. W-5, a chlorine-deficient
analogue of W-7 that interacts only weakly with calmodulin (23,26),
did not inhibit enzyme release from human PMNs. These results are
explained on the basis of known different affinities to calmodulin
of W-7 and W-5, thus supporting the notion that W-7 is acting as a
specific calmodulin antagonist.

        Human platelets possess granules containing a variety of medi-
ators and enzymatic systems. Recent evidence supports the hypothesis
that chemical mediators released from human platelets following immunological activation and aggregation might play a significant role
in inflammation and during allergic reactions (27). We therefore
studied the effects of several calmodulin antagonists on human platelet aggregation induced by several stimuli (ADP, thrombin, collagen,
and adrenaline). Figure 2 shows the effect of TFP on ADP-induced
platelet aggregation. TFP inhibited dose dependently ADP-induced
platelet aggregation. Similar results were obtained when aggregation
was induced by adrenaline, thrombin, and collagen and when W-7 was
used (25). By contrast, TFP sulfoxide, a compound which has low affinity for calmodulin (18), did not inhibit platelet aggregation.

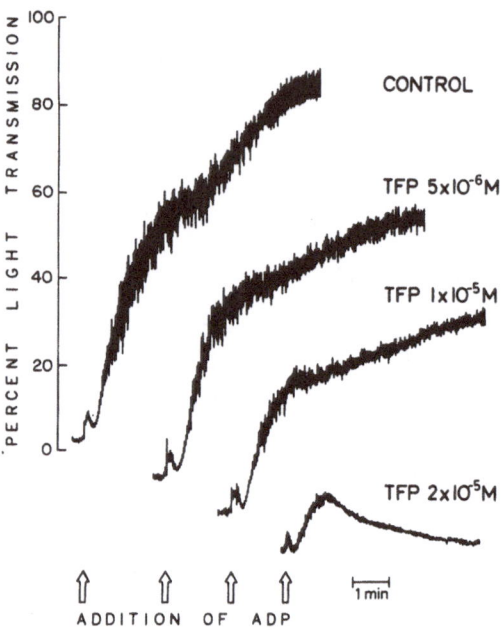

Fig. 2.   Dose response curves of inhibition of ADP-induced human
          platelet aggregation by trifluoperazine dihydrochloride

These data indicate that two different calmodulin antagonists,
such as TFP and W-7, at concentrations that effectively antagonize
calmodulin effects, inhibit histamine release from basophils and
enzyme release from PMNs induced by several immunological and non-
immunological stimuli. Furthermore, our data show that TFP and W-7
inhibit human platelet aggregation induced by a variety of stimuli.
Previous studies have demonstrated that both TFP and W-7 are spe-
c'´ic inhibitors of calmodulin-activated enzymes and calmodulin-
mediated processes (20,23,25). The presence of this protein in human
inflammatory cells has been demonstrated (3,28) and it is now well
established that calmodulin plays a pivoting role in cellular regulation (1). Our results indicating that two specific calmodulin antagonists are potent inhibitors of the secretory response of human
basophils and PMNs support the hypothesis that this protein is involved in the control of the release of preformed mediators from
human inflammatory cells.

Histamine secretion from human basophils and enzyme release
from PMNs are dependent upon the intracellular Ca^{2+} and cylic AMP
concentration (13,14), the state of microtubule assembly, and the
activation of phospholipase A_2 (13,15). Calmodulin is a ubiquitous
and versatile Ca^{2+}-binding protein that controls all these enzymes
and cellular functions. In fact, calmodulin has been reported to

stimulate phospholipase A_2 activity and TFP has been found to inhibit this stimulation (8). In addition, it has been demonstrated that TFP inhibits human platelet secretion and aggregation by blocking the activation of phospholipase A_2 (9). Therefore, it is likely that TFP and W-7 inhibit the secretory processes of human basophils and PMNs and platelet aggregation by interacting with calmodulin and influencing some of the calmodulin-dependent enzymes. Our previous results indicate that stimulation of specific surface receptor on human inflammatory cells, or the intracellular translocation of Ca^{2+}, activate phospholipase A_2 which plays an essential role in the control of both histamine release and lysosomal enzymes secretion (15,17). Therefore, it is possible that TFP and W-7 bind to calmodulin and block its ability to activate phospholipase A_2 following basophil, PMNs and platelet stimulation.

Finally, from a pharmacological point of view, it is possible to speculate that a specific inhibitor of calmodulin in human inflammatory cells, by blocking basophil and PMN secretion and platelet aggregation, will provide a new basis for the treatment of human inflammatory disorders.

ACKNOWLEDGEMENT

Supported in part by grants 80.00501.05 and 81.00272.04 from the C.N.R. (Rome, Italy).

REFERENCES

1. Cheung, W.Y., Science 207:19 (1980).
2. Means, A.R., Tash, J.S. and Chafouleas, J.G., Physiol. Rev. 62:1 (1982).
3. Jones, H.P., Ghai, G., Petrone, W.F. and McCord, J.M., Biochim. Biophys. Acta 714:152 (1982).
4. Chafouleas, J.G., Dedman, J.R., Munjaal, R.P. and Means, A.R., J. Biol. Chem. 254:10262 (1979).
5. Takeshige, K. and Minakami, S., Biochem. Biophys. Res. Comm. 99:484 (1981).
6. Weiss, B., Fertel, R., Figlin, R. and Uzunov, P., Mol. Pharmacol. 10:615 (1974).
7. Wolff, J., Cook, G.H., Goldhammer, A.R. and Berkowitz, S.A., Proc. Natl. Acad. Sci. USA 77:3841 (1980).
8. Wong, P.Y-K. and Cheung, W.Y., Biochem. Biophys. Res. Comm. 90:473 (1979).
9. Walenga, R.W., Opas, E.E. and Feinstein, M.B., J. Biol. Chem. 256:12523 (1981).
10. Means, A.R. and Dedman, J.R., Nature 285:73 (1980).
11. Lee, Y.C. and Wolff, J., J. Biol. Chem. 257:6306 (1982).

12. Marone, G., Kagey-Sobotka, A. and Lichtenstein, L.M., J. Immunol. 123:1669 (1979).

13. Marone, G., Plaut, M. and Lichtenstein, L.M., in: "Respiratory Allergy"(Eds. G. Melillo, G. D'Amato, G. Cocco and M. Ceccucci) Masson, p. 109 (1980).

14. Marone, G., Findlay, S.R. and Lichtenstein, L.M., J. Immunol. 123:1473 (1979).

15. Marone, G., Kagey-Sobotka, A. and Lichtenstein, L.M., Clin. Immunol. Immunopathol. 20:231 (1981).

16. Marone, G., Thomas, L.L. and Lichtenstein, L.M., J. Immunol. 125:2277 (1980).

17. Marone, G. and Condorelli, M., Fed. Proc. 40:1024 (1981).

18. Levin, R.M. and Weiss, B., Biochim. Biophys. Acta. 540:197 (1978).

19. Hidaka, H., Yamaki, T., Naka, M., Tanaka, T., Hayashi, H. and Kobayashi, R., Molec. Pharmacol. 17:66 (1980).

20. Weiss, B., Prozialek, W., Cimino, M., Barnette, M.S. and Wallace, T.L., Ann. N. Y. Acad. Sci. 356:319 (1980).

21. Levin, R.M. and Weiss, B., Molec. Pharmacol. 13:690 (1977).

22. Hidaka, H., Yamaki, T., Totsuka, T. and Asano, M., Mol. Pharmacol. 15:49 (1979).

23. Hidaka, H., Sasaki, Y., Tanaka, T., Endo, T., Ohno, S., Fujii, Y. and Nagata, T., Proc. Natl. Acad. Sci. 78:4354 (1981).

24. Kanamori, M., Naka, M., Asano, M. and Hidaka, H., J. Pharmacol. Exp. Ther. 217:494 (1981).

25. Nishikawa, M., Tanaka, T. and Hidaka, H., Nature 287:863 (1980).

26. Asano, M., Suzuki, Y. and Hidaka, H., J. Pharmacol. Exp. Ther. 220:191 (1982).

27. Knawer, K.A., Lichtenstein, L.M., Adkinson, N.F.Jr. and Fish, J.E., New Engl. J. Med. 304:1404 (1981).

28. Young, N., Gergely, P. and Crawford, N., Eur. J. Biochem. 120:303 (1981).

CONTRIBUTORS

Arnon, R. Department of Chemical Immunology, The Weizmann
    Institute of Science, Rehovot 76100, Israel

Atfield, G. Department of Immunology, The London Hospital
    Medical School, University of London, London E1 2AD, UK

Ballieux, R.E. Department of Clinical Immunology, University Hospital,
    Utrecht, The Netherlands

Ben-Nun, A. Department of Cell Biology, The Weizmann
    Institute of Science, Rehovot, Israel

Berkel, A.I. Immunology Unit, Institute of Child Health,
    Hacettepe University, Ankara, Turkey

Bianco, P. Department of Medicine, II School of Medicine,
    University of Naples, 80131 Napoli, Italy

Bohn, A. Lehrstuhl für Medizinische Mikrobiologie und Immunologie,
    Ruhr-Universitat Bochum, FRG

Borgeat, P. Départment d'Endocrinologie Moléculaire,
    Le Centre de L-Université Laval, SteFoye, Quebec, Canada

Bottazzo, G.F. Department of Immunology, Middlesex
    Hospital Medical School, London W1, UK

Bremm, K. Lehrstuhl für Medizinische Mikrobiologie und Immunologie,
    Ruhr-Universität Bochum, FRG

Bud, H. Laboratory of Gene Structure and Expression,
    National Institute for Medical Research, The Ridgeway,
    Mill Hill, London NW7 1AA, UK

Bullman, H. Laboratory of Gene Structure and Expression,
    National Institute for Medical Research, The Ridgeway,
    Mill Hill, London NW7 1AA, UK

Cabellero, F. Departments of Pediatrics and Medicine,
   University of Colorado Health Sciences Center,
   Denver, Colorado 80262, USA

Canegrati, A. Istituto di Richerche Farmacologiche
   "Mario Negri" 20157 Milano, Italy

Ciliv, G. Immunology Unit, Institute of Child Health,
   Hacettepe University, Ankara, Turkey

Cohen, I.R. Department of Cell Biology, The Weizmann
   Institute, Rehovot, Israel

Columbo, M. Department of Medicine, II School of Medicine,
   University of Naples, 80131 Napoli, Italy

Condorelli, M. Department of Medicine, II School of Medicine,
   University of Naples, 80131 Napoli, Italy

Crea, A.E.G. Institut für Organische Chemie, Universität
   Düsseldorf, FRG

Czitrom, A.A. ICRF Tumour Immunology Unit, University College London,
   London, UK

Domdey, H. Department of Molecular Biology, Swiss
   Institute for Experimental Cancer Research, CH 1066
   Epalinges, Switzerland

Doniach, D. Department of Immunology, Middlesex
   Hospital Medical School, London W1, UK

Edwards, S. ICRF Tumour Immunology Unit, University College London,
   London, UK

Erb, P. Institute for Microbiology, University of Basel,
   Basel, Switzerland

Ersoy, F. Immunology Unit, Institute of Child Health,
   Hacettepe University, Ankara, Turkey

Falsone, G. Institut für Organische Chemie, Universität
   Düsseldorf, FRG

Feldmann, M. ICRF Tumour Immunology Unit, University College London,
   London, UK

Ferluga, J. Department of Immunology, The London Hospital
   Medical School, University of London, London E1 2AD, UK

Festenstein, H. Department of Immunology, The London
    Hospital Medical School, University of London,
    London E1 2AD, UK

Fey, G. Department of Molecular Biology, Swiss Institute
    for Experimental Cancer Research, CH 1066 Epalinges, Switzerland

Flavell, R. Laboratory of Gene Structure and Expression,
    National Institute for Medical Research, The Ridgeway,
    Mill Hill, London NW7 1AA, UK

Flood, P.M. Department of Pathology, The Howard Hughes
    Medical Institute for Cellular Immunology, Yale
    University School of Medicine, New Haven, Connecticut 06510, USA

Gershon, R.K. (deceased) Department of Pathology, The Howard Hughes
    Medical Institute for Cellular Immunology, Yale
    University School of Medicine, New Haven, Connecticut 06510, USA

Golden, L. Laboratory of Gene Structure and Expression,
    National Institute for Medical Research, The Ridgeway,
    Mill Hill, London NW7 1AA, UK

Hardt, C. Institut für Medical Mikrobiologie, Universität
    Mainz, 6500 Mainz, FRG

Harrison, R.A. Medical Research Council Centre, Cambridge, UK

Hauptmann, G. Institut d'Hématologie and Centre de
    Transfusion Sanguine, Strasbourg, France

Hayward, A.R. Departments of Pediatrics and Medicine,
    University of Colorado Health Sciences Center,
    Denver, Colorado 80262, USA

Heijnen, C.J. Department of Clinical Immunology,
    University Children's Hospital "Het Wilhelmina Kinderziekenhuis",
    Utrecht, The Netherlands

Hohlfeld, R. Neurological University Hospital, Düsseldorf, FRG

Hurst, J. Laboratory of Gene Structure and Expression,
    National Institute for Medical Research, The Ridgeway,
    Mill Hill, London NW7 1AA, UK

James, R.F.L. ICRF Tumour Immunology Unit, University College,
    London WC1E 6BT, UK

Kabat, E.A. Departments of Microbiology, Human Genetics and
    Development, and Neurology, and the Cancer Center,
    Columbia University College of Physicians and Surgeons,
    New York 10032, USA

Kalies, I. Institute of Clinical Immunology, University,
    Erlangen, FRG

Katz, D.R. ICRF Tumour Immunology Unit, University College
    London, London, UK

Kazmaier, M. Department of Molecular Biology, Swiss
    Institute for Experimental Cancer Research, CH 1066
    Epalinges, Switzerland

Kohler, P. Departments of Pediatrics and Medicine,
    University of Colorado Health Sciences Center,
    Denver, Colorado 80262, USA

König, W. Lehrstuhl für Medizinische Mikrobiologie und Immunologie,
    Ruhr-Universität Bochum, FRG

Krönke, M. Institut für Medizinische Mikrobiologie,
    Universität Mainz, 6500 Mainz, FRG

Krumwieh, D. Max-Planck-Institut für Immunobiologie,
    D-7800 Freiburg, FRG

Kuis, W. University Children's Hospital, Utrecht, The Netherlands

Lachmann, P.J. Medical Research Counsil Centre, Cambridge, UK

Lang, H. Max-Planck-Institut für Immunobiologie,
    D-7800 Freiburg, FRG

Leben, L. Department of Immunology, The London Hospital
    Medical School, University of London, London E1 2AD, UK

Lohmann-Matthes, M.L. Max-Planck-Institut für Immunobiologie,
    D-7800, Freiburg, FRG

Louie, D. Department of Pathology, The Howard Hughes Medical
    Institute for Cellular Immunology Yale University
    School of Medicine, New Haven, Connecticut 06510, USA

Luini, W. Istituto di Richerche Farmacologiche "Mario Negri",
    20157 Milano, Italy

Marone, G. Department of Medicine, II School of Medicine,
    University of Naples, 80131 Napoli, Italy

Matter, A. Immunology Laboratories France, Schering-Plough Corporation,
    69572 Dardilly, France

Mellor, A.L. Laboratory of Gene Structure and Expression,
    National Institute for Medical Research, The Ridgeway,
    Mill Hill, London NW7 1AA, UK

Merendino, A. Istituto di Richerche Farmacologiche "Mario Negri"
    20157 Milano, Italy

Müller, V. Department of Molecular Biology, Swiss Institute for
    Experimental Cancer Research, CH 1066 Epalinges, Switzerland

Olsson, L. Medical Department A, State University Hospital,
    Copenhagen, Denmark

Parish, W.E. Environmental Safety Laboratory, Unilever Research,
    Colworth House, Sharnbrook, Bedford MK44 1LQ, UK

Pasqualetto, E. Istituto di Richerche Farmacologiche "Mario Negri"
    20157 Milano, Italy

Pereira, T.A.E. Division of Immunology, Clinical Research Centre,
    Harrow, Middlesex, UK

Pfeiffer, Ph. Lehrstuhl für Medizinische Mikrobiologie und Immunologie,
    Ruhr-Universität Bochum, FRG

Pfizenmaier, K. Institut für Medizinische Mikrobiologie,
    Universitat Mainz, 6500 Mainz, FRG

Platts-Mills, T.A.E. Division of Allergy and Clinical Immunology,
    Department of Medicine, University of Virginia, Charlottesville,
    Virginia 22908, USA

Poto, S. Department of Medicine, II School of Medicine, University
    of Naples, 80131 Napoli, Italy

Ramila, G. Institute for Microbiology, University of Basel,
    Basel, Switzerland

Rijkers, G.T. University Children's Hospital, Utrecht,
    The Netherlands

Röllinghoff, M. Institut für Medizinische Mikrobiologie,
    Universität Mainz, 6500 Mainz, FRG

Romano, M. Istituto di Richerche Farmacologiche "Mario Negri",
    20157 Milano, Italy

Roord, J.J. University Children's Hospital, Utrecht, The Netherlands

Sanal, Ö. Immunology Unit, Institute of Child Health,
    Hacettepe University, Ankara, Turkey

Sanderson, A.R. MRC Immunology Team, Nag's Head Yard Medical School,
    Guy's Hospital, London SE1 9RT, UK

Santamaria, M. Department of Immunology, The London Hospital
    Medical School, University of London, London E1 2AD, UK

Schalke, B.C.G. Clinical Research Unit for Multiple Sclerosis,
    Max-Planck-Society, D-8700 Würzburg, FRG

Scheurich, P. Institut für Medizinische Mikrobiologie, Universität
    Mainz, 6500 Mainz, FRG

Simpson, E. Clinical Research Centre, Watford Road, Harrow
    Middlesex HA1 3UJ, UK

Sironi, M. Istituto di Richerche Farmacologiche "Mario Negri"
    20157 Milano, Italy

Sklenar, I. Institute for Microbiology, University of Basel,
    Basel, Switzerland

Southgate, C. Department of Molecular Biology, Swiss Institute
    for Experimental Cancer Research, CH 1066 Epalinges, Switzerland

Spaapen, L.J.M. University Children's Hospital, Utrecht,
    The Netherlands

Spreafico, F. Istituto di Richerche Farmacologiche "Mario Negri"
    20157 Milano, Italy

Spur, B. Institut für Organische Chemie, Universität Düsseldorf, FRG

Stern, A. Institute for Microbiology, University of Basel,
    Basel, Switzerland

Stockinger, H. Institut für Medizinische Mikrobiologie,
    Universität Mainz, 6500 Mainz, FRG

Stoop, J.W. University Children's Hospital, Utrecht, The Netherlands

Sun, D. Max-Planck-Institut für Immunobiologie, D-7800 Freiburg, FRG

Sunshine, G.H. ICRF Tumour Immunology Unit, University College
    London, London, UK

Szperalski, B. Lehrstuhl für Medizinische Mikrobiologie und
   Immunologie, Ruhr-Universität Bochum, FRG

Taylor, P.M. Division of Immunology, National Institute for
   Medical Research, The Ridgeway, Mill Hill, London NW7 1AA, UK

Termijtelen, A. Department of Immunohaematology and Blood Bank,
   University Hospital, 2333 AA Leiden, The Netherlands

Theobald, K. Lehrstuhl für Medizinische Mikrobiologie und Immunologie,
   Ruhr-Universität Bochum, FRG

Townsend, A.R.M. Division of Immunology, National Institute for
   Medical Research, The Ridgeway, Mill Hill, London NW7 1AA, UK

van Leeuwen, A. Department of Immunohaematology and Blook Bank,
   University Hospital, 2333 AA Leiden, The Netherlands

van Rood, J.J. Department of Immunohaematology and Blook Bank,
   University Hospital, 2333 AA Leiden, The Netherlands

Vecchi, A. Istituto di Richerche Farmacologiche "Mario Negri"
   20157, Milano, Italy

Wagner, H. Institut für Medizinische Mikrobiologie, Universität
   Mainz, 6500 Mainz, FRG

Webster, A.D.B. Division of Immunology, Clinical Research Centre,
   Harrow, Middlesex, UK

Weiss, E. Laboratory of Gene Structure and Expression, National
   Institute for Medical Research, The Ridgeway, Mill Hill,
   London NW7 1AA, UK

Wekerle, H. Clinical Research Unit for Multiple Sclerosis, Max-
   Planck-Society, D-8700 Würzburg, FRG

Wielbauer, H. Department of Molecular Biology, Swiss Institute
   for Experimental Cancer Research, CH 1066 Epalinges, Switzerland

Wilkins, S.R. Division of Immunology, Clinical Research Centre,
   Harrow, Middlesex, UK

Yeğin, O. Immunology Unit, Institute of Child Health,
   Hacettepe University, Ankara, Turkey

Zegers, B.J.M. University Children's Hospital, Utrecht,
   The Netherlands

INDEX